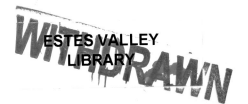

HEALING

ALSO BY THERESA BROWN

The Shift: One Nurse, Twelve Hours, Four Patients' Lives

*Critical Care: A New Nurse Faces Death, Life,
and Everything in Between*

HEALING

When a Nurse Becomes a Patient

THERESA BROWN, RN

ALGONQUIN BOOKS
OF CHAPEL HILL 2022

Published by
Algonquin Books of Chapel Hill
Post Office Box 2225
Chapel Hill, North Carolina 27515-2225

a division of
Workman Publishing
225 Varick Street
New York, New York 10014

Library of Congress Cataloging-in-Publication Data
Names: Brown, Theresa, author.
Title: Healing : when a nurse becomes a patient / Theresa Brown, RN.
Description: First edition. | Chapel Hill, North Carolina : Algonquin
Books of Chapel Hill, 2022. | Includes bibliographical references. |
Summary: "When a cancer nurse becomes a cancer patient, she has to
confront the most critical, terrified, sometimes furious patient she's
ever encountered: herself. A frank look at struggling with illness while
navigating the health care maze"— Provided by publisher.
Identifiers: LCCN 2021052738 | ISBN 9781643750699 (hardcover) |
ISBN 9781643752969 (ebook)
Subjects: LCSH: Brown, Theresa,—Health. | Breast—Cancer—Patients—
Biography. | Women nurses—Biography. Classification: LCC RC280.B8
B7464 2022 | DDC 616.99/4490092 [B]—dc23/eng/20211124
LC record available at https://lccn.loc.gov/2021052738

10 9 8 7 6 5 4 3 2 1
First Edition

In Memory of Sharon

Disclaimer

This book is a work of memory, though the memories surrounding my cancer diagnosis and treatment are sometimes sharp, sometimes blurred, sometimes nonexistent. Make of that what you choose. All names and initials are changed, just because, except for Sue Larson. You'll see why when you read that chapter.

CONTENTS

PART FOUR: THE LONG HAUL

HEALING

PROLOGUE

I WAS READING *Bad Feminist* by Roxane Gay the day I went for my scan. The inside cover of the book is neon pink—not the girlish pink of Disney princesses and bubble gum, but a knowing, winking pink. The color of a bad, as in badass, feminist: the kind of person who reads *Bad Feminist* while waiting for a mammogram.

It was a follow-up. I had mentioned it to my husband, Arthur, who was out of town, but no one else. I always got called back. Well, not always, but often, and I'd sweated the "need for additional screening" enough times that I had convinced myself there's no value to being anxious in advance.

I had a mammogram and an ultrasound: right side only. I waited calmly in the hallway in between the two scans, and then I waited in the ultrasound room after the tech left and before the radiologist came in. I might have wondered why the tech left, but instead I read my neon pink book, word by word, without knowing what I was reading.

A questionable scan merits an on-the-spot reading by an on-site radiologist, who came in and redid the ultrasound. She took a long time, which annoyed me, and then, once I considered why she might be slow, scared me. Finally she said, "I see a mass." A mass. I saw her in profile, gray hair pulled back from her face, her eyes focused on the screen.

It might seem like she could have said more, but those four words were already too many. I didn't move, speak, or sit up, but I did begin to cry, slowly. Tears dribbled out of each eye and slid down the sides of my face as I lay, silent, on the exam table.

I'm a former oncology nurse and a hospice nurse. I knew the importance of letting the doctor finish the scan, that panicking wouldn't help me or her as she took final measurements or did whatever she had to do. I figured I was knowledgeable enough about having cancer because I knew about specific cancers, that I understood cancer patients' feelings because I'd cared for so many, that I'd confronted mortality because I'd had a number of patients die. But I was wrong. Other people's mortality is categorically different from one's own. Actual mortality—which is to say, mine—had never, before this moment, seemed real.

"Could it be a fibroid adenoma?" I blurted out. I'd had those before and they're not cancerous.

"No," she said, gently shaking her head. "This looks ugly." She left, and as soon as I heard the door latch, I sat up and sobbed, my whole body shaking. Fear had found me and everything seemed upside down. My nurse-self had abandoned me and I had become a patient. Not just any kind of patient, either, but a cancer patient.

The ultrasound tech came back into the room so quietly I didn't hear her, but suddenly her arms were around me. She put her arms around me, a stranger, and said, "They can cure this." But that was what *I* did: comforted strangers.

Not even a day had passed since I started my testing. It was still sunny and a little colder than normal for September, but I had changed. The nurse was lost on the bottom, the patient flailing on the top. I was terrified and sad and angry. I was afraid and forlorn and enraged. I was frightened and bereft and irate. And that was just the beginning.

PART ONE

Who Am I?

ONE

Day One

MY FIRST DAY as a nurse, no one seemed to be expecting me. My preceptor—the nurse teaching me the job—showed up late. We had been told in our student clinicals that arriving late to the hospital was an unforgivable sin, but my preceptor didn't seem to care, or realize I was coming that day, and it took a while for her to get organized. They'd given her an extra, fifth, patient, plus me, and she grumbled about the combination. An older Black woman, she had a generous smile and was deliberative in almost everything she did. She also moved unhurriedly. Quick of step, and impatient to get on with learning the job, I muttered to myself about her slowness.

A few months later, as I began to really understand how to do the job, I realized my preceptor was one of the best nurses I ever worked with, but I couldn't see it right then. Time was of the essence, I thought. Speed mattered. I was good at moving fast, at juggling, making quick decisions about which problem to solve first. This was the training of motherhood in addition to nursing. I had baby twins and a toddler in my early thirties. When the twins turned one, I noted: "One year down and no missing limbs."

From Carrie P.—that was my preceptor's name—I learned that sometimes in nursing it takes time to notice what is really going on. "You look whicky-whacky," she would say to a patient askew in a bed. We would help the patient sit up, straighten the blankets, fluff the pillows, and a human being would emerge from the pile of linen. Then we could fully see that person.

A blinking call light outside a patient's room always drew Carrie P. That's how it's supposed to be, but often not how it is. Once it was a man having trouble peeing. He needed help standing upright—he couldn't urinate sitting down. He was weak, though, and even when he stood up, it took time for him to get all his urine out. Carrie P. and I braced him, one of us on each side, holding him up. She also held the plastic urinal and talked with him, giving encouragement and making small talk as if we were all meeting over coffee. In my head the minutes ticked by, but Carrie P. showed me how considered, hands-on care gives patients respect. She never finished her shifts on time and always strove for the ideal, even though it took me awhile to recognize that.

Carrie P. had a last name, of course, but she was always just "Carrie P." There must have been another Carrie at some point and the "P" became her differentiator. It stuck. There was no other nurse like her on the floor: so careful with patients' humanity, so clinically knowledgeable. We got along well, but one chaotic day we drew blood to prep a patient for a test and I used the wrong color tubes. She came so close to losing her patience: "I specifically told you to draw a blue and a yellow." I felt ashamed and stupid. The next shift I apologized for the mix-up. "Things like that happen," she said, neutral, focused on our work for the coming day. In that moment I saw that Carrie P. cared about the job more than anything else, more than hurrying, more than scolding a new nurse, and I felt grateful to have her as my preceptor.

But Carrie P. usually worked nights, and my manager wanted me to train during daylight exclusively because day shift was much busier than night shift and I would learn more. I was assigned another preceptor, M, who came from white, working-class Pittsburgh. M asked me about my PhD in English, whether I had kids, and why I chose to work with cancer patients. She seemed to dislike all three of my answers and we never clicked. My manager had worked as a nurse on the floor before her promotion and a group of nurses, including my new preceptor, were still close with her. I didn't understand that navigating the cliques on the floor would be central to succeeding there and I misjudged how powerful the bonds in those cliques were. I also had no idea how mean nurses could be to other nurses, that there was a tradition of nurses "eating their young."

My new preceptor had an aunt who had died of cancer. It gave her a personal connection to the disease and she revealed it with what seemed to me a trace of sanctimony. Sometimes I think about my response to M's third question: why did I choose oncology? I had been matter-of-fact. I said the science was really interesting and that there was a lot of cancer in my mother's family. I'm not sure why I was so curt and analytical—I could have easily revealed more, since my family history of cancer is extensive. My maternal grandmother had four cancers: breast, uterine, colon, and skin. Three maternal aunts had breast cancer, and one died from the disease when it spread to her brain. A maternal uncle died of colon cancer. I could have bonded with M over our shared family grief, but I didn't. My mother's siblings were not close and her mother died when I was very young. I didn't feel sad about their deaths from cancer. I feared the volume of cases among my relatives.

At that time, I told myself that I was fascinated by cancer, while being scared of it. A malignancy is impressively aggressive, biologically speaking. Cancer survives through stealth, taking nutrients and blood away from normal tissue, crowding healthy organs as it grows, invading other sites in the body. It presents as a relentless perversion of social Darwinism: cancer is not "fit," but it will survive, even if that means consuming the body that gives it life. We might call cancer cells an apex of evolution in that they adapt, often quickly, to stay alive, sometimes even becoming invulnerable to chemotherapy. That is why chemo regimens may include first-, second-, and third-line treatments. The higher a patient goes up the list, the more successfully that person's cancer has resisted the drugs.

I could not have articulated all that to M, and it probably wouldn't have helped if I had. Nursing education is a complicated story. I had a college degree in nursing and M's degree was from a community college. And I had a PhD—in English, not nursing, but still. For some nurses, the difference between a two-year associate's degree from a community college and a four-year bachelor's degree feels huge and can create insecurity. Suggest to a group of nurses that all RNs should have bachelor's degrees and the hackles among nurses who attended community college understandably rise at the implication that some nurses are "better" than others by virtue of being "more educated." My PhD likely only made me seem educationally farther away from M, and my intellectual interest in cancer might have seemed odd and unwelcome.

M, I think, looked at nursing as something she was personally committed to, and with which she had a personal connection. My explanation of myself *to* myself then, when I began working as an oncology nurse, was not personal in that way. Though of course it was. The full truth—and why I chose to work specifically with liquid tumor patients, those ill with leukemias and lymphomas—was something I had carefully hidden away, but here it is: My mother is a survivor of hairy-cell leukemia. It's a rare cancer, and usually people die with it, not of it, but she had it for almost a decade until an effective chemotherapy treatment came along and cured her. It was a long time ago, before I got married, had kids, and became a nurse.

I had packed that story away in bubble wrap. Then I placed the bubble wrap, with the memory protected inside it, in a plain cardboard box. I had taped the box closed and moved it to that place in the human brain where memories go to hide. Three years after I became a nurse, when I was also a nurse-writer and on my way to speak at Yale University, I thought about why I had become an oncology nurse. I knew they would ask me that question at the lecture, and I wanted to have a good answer. As I looked out the window of the plane, taking in a wide view of clear blue sky, my carefully packed mental box opened all by itself. *Of course*, I thought. My work as a cancer nurse, taking care of leukemia patients, suddenly made sense. Everything suddenly made sense.

My mother had leukemia. If I had talked about my mom's cancer, the nurses on the floor might have identified with my struggle instead of minding about my education. Oncology nurses feel bad for family members of cancer patients, and in general, people hearing my mother's diagnosis would breathe in sharply, step back. The nurses on my floor would know that hairy cell leukemia is not the same disease as acute leukemia, but I think they would have had empathy for me anyway. It is terrible when anyone's mother has cancer.

There was no way I could have said any of that to M, my preceptor, because I didn't know it myself. I wonder, sometimes, if I had known that, and told M, our working relationship would have been easier. I wonder. I wonder if I had better understood nursing, and myself, whether I could have toughed it out in that first job, whether that in-group of nurse bullies would not have judged me as someone who didn't belong. It's impossible to say. Arguably, bullies are always looking for their next victim. That explains why no one welcomed me when I got there, why they overloaded Carrie P. on my first day, and why even Carrie P., who was so dedicated to others, kept aloof from the spite of the other nurses. Only later did I learn that the unit was notorious for treating new nurses, and the medical interns and residents, badly.

After six months, I left that job. The rule was, you had to remain in a position for a year before you could transfer, but I refused to take no for an answer and insisted on switching jobs earlier. It worked. I moved to another medical oncology unit. There were cliques and strong personalities on the new ward, too, which was separated by an elevator bay from the old one, but not to the same corrosive degree. No one was looking for a target.

Afterwards, one of the nurses' aides from the old floor asked me why I left. Then he answered his own question: "Too many bitches, right?" It was a gratifying answer, but likely untrue. Too many nurses unhappy, threatened, insecure, along with a manager who did nothing to make the problem go away. What does any of this have to do with cancer? Nothing, right? There are mean people everywhere. But maybe it's not that simple. Maybe some amalgam of suffering, sorrow, uncertainty, and, possibly, powerlessness in the face of all that, brought out the mean especially well among that set of nurses. We cured patients, but many also died, and sometimes the cures didn't stick, which was heartbreaking. Not all the nurses were able to accept, with grace, the ongoing tragedy of our work. And powerlessness was part of the problem, too, the kind of powerlessness that led a nurse, after a patient had died unexpectedly, to kick a chair across the nurses' station. She was the meanest nurse on the floor and, at that moment, hurting.

I became an oncology nurse without knowing why, then figured it out. Ideally, nursing is a sacred duty. It can be just a job, a steady paycheck, but the best nurses dedicate themselves to the work, for all kinds of different reasons.

The road of life can fork in such a way that we're unsure which path we're on, or why, but we keep going. That's survival. Cancer casts a long shadow, but I've been living in it my entire life. That's survival, too.

TWO

Rage

THE PATIENT WAS nineteen. That's young to be on an adult hospital floor, young to have his particular cancer. He'd grown up in rural Pennsylvania, and being stuck in a hospital room kept him at a low simmer. It wasn't his first hospital stay, and it would not be his last.

That shift, on the new floor, where we did bone-marrow transplants, it was my job, as his nurse, to send him home after his blood transfusion finished.

His mother was also there. She was also a nurse, but mostly a mother when I met her in her son's hospital room. Her full, straight bangs and bleached blond hair that stopped just at her shoulders made an impression of curated control. But waiting for her son's hospital discharge had put her at a low simmer, too. I could tell from her compressed lips, the way she sat forward in her chair and watched everything I did. Neither of them said much to me, but every time I walked into the room, I felt their anger. I felt it so much that I dreaded going into his room, but I had to. I needed to get him ready to go home.

When the transfusion finished, another nurse came into the room with me to do a required double-check. Our hospital floor was testing a new kind of needleless connector, called a cap, that went on the ends of the intravenous catheters that had been surgically implanted into, and protruded out of, our patients' chests. The caps were flimsy and broke apart easily.

I knew the transfusion had ended because the bag of blood hanging from the IV pole, connected to the patient via special filtered tubing, was empty. I disconnected the blood tubing from the "permanent" IV line attached to the patient and threw the empty bag of blood away. Then I used alcohol to clean the end of the permanent line, and injected 10 mL of saline into it to clear the line of any blood left over from the transfusion. I twisted the now-empty saline syringe off the end of the patient's implanted IV line, and as I did that, the IV cap came apart. Its interior piece of hard blue plastic, about one inch long, fell onto the floor.

The cap was a barrier against infection and had to be replaced right away. I took a new cap out of my pocket and screwed it onto the end of the patient's attached IV catheter. Meanwhile, the nurse who had come into the room with me verified on the computer that the right unit of blood had been transfused into the right patient. She finished, I finished, and the patient, who had been sitting on the bed, his torso tensed like a spring in a jack-in-the-box, stood up, putting his whole weight on the piece of blue plastic that had fallen to the floor.

He was barefoot—ouch—and he swore elaborately. He accused me of not knowing how to do my job. "This one thing," he kept saying, meaning the cap. If I couldn't get this one thing right, if I couldn't pick things up from the floor when it mattered, how could I get anything right?

I apologized, and I meant it, but it made no difference. So, I stood there, taking it. From my point of view, he was entitled. To have cancer at such a young age, and to have his nurse, the professional meant to look out for him, cause him pain . . . I waited, saying nothing, until he stopped. Then I squatted down and picked the piece of blue plastic off the floor. It had a surprisingly sharp edge. It would hurt to step on it. I cradled it in the palm of my hand, and the other nurse and I left the room.

"You handled that just the right way," she said once we were outside the room. "Not to say anything, not to defend yourself." She waved one hand in the air, swatting away useless explanations.

"Hey, thanks," I said. What she told me, including the hand gestures—it helped.

I threw the piece of blue plastic away. Damn those cheap caps. Damn. And I still had to go back in the room to officially discharge him. And his IV line dressing—the bandage that covered where the implanted intravenous line entered his chest—needed to be changed before he left.

His discharge paperwork took longer to prepare than it should have, which is typical, but frustrating. Finally I had it and I went into the room. I felt the patient's and his mother's anger again, stronger, sharp now. I went through his instructions, reading off medications, outlining his follow-up care, trying not to hurry while wanting to hurry. His mother's lips, pressed tautly together, maybe held back the abuse she wanted to inflict on me, on us, her son's caregivers, to equalize the pain that cancer inflicted on him, and her. It wasn't personal— I knew that—but then again, I was the person in the room with them.

Just as they were getting ready to leave, I remembered that the bandage over the patient's intravenous line needed to be replaced. Every seven days, each patient gets a new dressing, and it's a bit of a rigmarole because the procedure has to be sterile. The patient and his mother, however, were packed and standing up, ready to go. His mother, a nurse, had changed the dressing herself at home when needed, so I gave them a choice: I could change the dressing right then, delaying them slightly, or she could change it when they got home. She shrugged. Then without looking at me she said, "I'll do it." And they left.

A few days later my manager called me into her office. The patient had come to an outpatient appointment at the cancer center across the street with the old dressing—the one I should have changed—still in place. Nothing bad happened as a result, but I had broken a rule and someone had reported me.

I said that the patient's mother had offered to change the dressing herself, that they were in an incredible hurry to get out of the hospital. My manager understood, but told me I should have written a note detailing the patient's choice.

I wondered why the patient's mother didn't change the dressing. Maybe once she got home she was too busy, or too tired, or both. Maybe they had run out of in-home supplies and she thought I wouldn't give her more because that's what the rules say, even though nurses, including me, gave out extra supplies all the time. Maybe she wanted to be her son's mom and not his nurse during their brief time at home. It doesn't matter—there were no negative sequelae—but of course I should have made a note in the chart specifying that the patient's mother planned to change the dressing at home. Truth is, I never thought of it. After they left, I only wanted to be done with them. I had looked his anger right in the face, and then, as soon as I could, I looked away.

WHEN I RECEIVED my own diagnosis from the radiologist, who never said cancer, only "a mass," even the firm, enveloping hug from the ultrasound tech and her assurance that "they can cure this" couldn't stop my crying.

I got parked in a hallway to wait for an additional mammogram. Now that the ultrasound had revealed a problem, they wanted to rescan part of my breast using mammography. Other women waiting for their own mammograms were seated near me as I quietly cried. It was the same hallway where I had waited before, and I felt exposed, but mostly I felt guilty. I figured that every woman there knew why I was crying and would prefer not to be reminded that her day, like mine, might include being diagnosed with breast cancer.

The mammography tech (not the comforting ultrasound tech) called me for the new mammogram and I kept crying. Slow tears, one after another, slid down my face while the tech squeezed and flattened my right breast between clear plastic plates. I held my breath and let it out; the tech asked me to step back and reposition, and squeezed and flattened my right breast with the plates again. The tears never stopped falling, so patiently, one right after another. When the mammogram was over, before she sent me back to the hallway, the tech said, "I hope everything turns out OK." I looked at her, then walked out.

Afterwards the ultrasound tech who had been so comforting when I burst into tears led me into a darkened room. The walls were covered with outsize computer screens glowing in black and white. "We live in the dark," explained the radiologist, seated in front of a large monitor. She showed me the mass in my right breast. It was small and irregular, pointy like a star. Except it wasn't a star. It was, possibly, the beginning of the end of my life. The diagnosis was not 100 percent at this point. Only a sample of tissue, from a biopsy, would reveal whether I definitely had cancer.

Still, I cried steadily. When the tears hit my chin, I wiped them away with the back of my hand. "I can't stop crying," I said.

"It's the ones who don't react that I worry about," the radiologist said, still looking at the mass—my mass—on the screen. "I worry that they haven't heard what I've said."

I returned to the dressing room and the kind ultrasound tech gave me a psalm she had written down, a message about heavenly protection. I thanked her. I hugged her. "They can cure this," she reminded me, and then told me that she likely had something incurable herself; a final test result would soon confirm her diagnosis. I didn't know what to say. I couldn't take it in. But hearing it reminded me there's all kinds of pain in the world, and I stopped crying.

In the dressing room I took off the wrap-around pink cotton gown I'd put on a few hours before and put back on my shirt and sweater. My outfit—a long sweater and black leggings I'd worn that morning to make me look tough and strong—no longer communicated anything other than *these are my clothes*. My book, *Bad Feminist*, seemed the work of an alien. I picked up my purse and put my pink gown in the bin for dirty laundry.

After leaving the dressing room, I sat down at the registration desk inside the waiting area. The radiologist had assured me that I wouldn't leave the hospital without an appointment for a biopsy.

I perched in the chair, shoulders hunched forward, aware of the tear lines streaking my face. There was a computer on the desk and an empty chair behind it, but no one came to schedule my biopsy, which I needed to confirm the diagnosis. Finally, one of the receptionists spoke up. "She leaves at three," she said, gesturing towards the chair, "You just missed her."

I looked at my watch. It said three o'clock on the dot.

You just missed her.

Just missed her.

You just missed her.

No "Sorry" or "Call tomorrow morning after eight a.m." or "Let me see if she's actually gone."

Had no one told the scheduler that a patient needing a biopsy would be coming to the desk? Or did she know and leave anyway?

You just missed her.

Just. Missed. Her.

I wanted to slam the receptionist into the wall.

I wanted to punch her in the stomach and as she doubled over, gasping for breath, smash my fist into the bridge of her nose. I wanted to hear bone crack. I wanted to see blood, have her say *NO*, beg for mercy.

But, of course, none of that happened.

The next morning, early, I called the scheduler. The first biopsy appointment she gave me was two weeks away. "No," I said. Just no. And then I added, "The radiologist is 'very concerned.' This is the best you can do?"

Turns out they were short a radiologist due to a family emergency. She had spent all of the previous day "rearranging everyone else's schedule." Ah. That likely explained why she shut up shop at 2:59 p.m.

"That has nothing to do with me," I told her.

"Well, I know it doesn't," she said, with a slightly, only slightly, chastening tone. It was a Friday and she found me an appointment for the next Wednesday. It didn't even take that long. I thanked her sincerely, but this is what I did not say: Thank you thank you for doing your job today, when yesterday you had to straighten out everyone's schedule, while I, well, I just had this small problem of being diagnosed with breast cancer.

You just missed her.

We're short a radiologist. Short, short, short a radiologist.

You just missed her.

The experience grated. It stuck.

Like a small, sharp piece of blue plastic cutting into the tender skin of my sole.

THREE

Bob & Wendy

THEY WERE BOB and Wendy. She had fashionably cut short brown hair with bangs that curled just above her eyes. He had not much hair and was very tall.

He was the patient and she, the wife. He had a new diagnosis of acute leukemia. Usually when someone comes in as a "new leuk," they seem panic-stricken, and their partner (if they have one) seems lost, too. Not Bob and Wendy. Going into his room felt like being welcomed to a small, intimate party. Middle-aged and financially comfortable, he was the relaxed host who was always happy to see you, while she pumped energy into the room with her nonstop questions and quick smile that crinkled the skin around her eyes.

I was Bob's nurse on one of his first days in the hospital. Before leaving to go home, his night-shift nurse told me she had done her best to teach both of them about Bob's disease and treatment. "Lots and lots of patient education," she said. It's what she thought they needed.

I'd heard this before—teaching patients is important—but suddenly I understood how overwhelming it must be, how frightening. For our patients like Bob, a routine lab test, some tiredness, a bruise that wouldn't go away, led to blood work, the diagnosis of acute myelogenous leukemia, or AML, and an immediate hospital admission that would last at least six weeks. In the hospital, the patient and family would be bombarded with information, procedures, blood draws, nurses, doctors, mediocre food, and interrupted sleep. A surgeon would implant a central intravenous line that left tubes hanging out of the patient's chest. New medications, including chemotherapy, would begin and the patient would have to sleep, walk, go to the bathroom, and shower, all while connected to an IV pole on wheels.

This time, all the talking, the educating, struck me as too much too soon. I don't know what it was about Bob and Wendy, but I told them, "We're going to be telling you a lot of things over the next several days. Don't feel you need to remember all of it. Let it wash over you. In the end, you'll know more about treatment for leukemia than you ever wanted to."

They both nodded; they liked that. And Wendy smiled, her eyes crinkling again.

Something. There was something about them. Another time that day I went into his room and reacted in a way I never had before: I wanted to save them. Yes, not just him, but both of them. And to save them, I wanted a magic wand, not central lines and daily labs and chemo, but the stuff of fairy tales: magical godmothers, good witches, possibly a genie hiding in a lamp.

I felt that wish like a lump in my throat. I pictured the magic wand as a pinwheel, leaving a trail of animated stars in its wake as I waved it over them, making him well.

I tried to talk about this feeling with some of the other nurses. No one seemed to understand. Or maybe they understood too well. We're in the business of saving people, but we don't always save them.

BOB WE DID save—during that first stay—and then he came back for a stem cell transplant. When I walked in he said, "Hi, Theresa," without pause, as if I was a close friend he hadn't seen in a while, come by to say hello.

He was reading a book about fish. It might have been the bestseller *Four Fish*, but I think it was a different bestseller called *Cod: A Biography of the Fish that Changed the World.* Either way, I looked at it skeptically. I couldn't see reading a whole book about fish. I teased him about it, gently, and he said, oh no, then explained how interesting it was, how the story of fish is part of so many other stories. "You wouldn't expect that, but it's true," he said.

From what I saw, nothing disturbed his equilibrium. Nothing.

She was different. For one thing, she wasn't there that day, which was unusual. I heard through the grapevine that some of the other nurses thought that staying overnight with him in the hospital was wearing her down. Our manager had intervened, encouraging Wendy to go home to sleep, or at least take a shower, maybe work in her garden, be separate for a time.

They differed in their approach to his illness, also. He wanted to be told what treatments he needed and when they would happen and he refused any more information after that. She wanted to know everything: Why *x* instead of *y*? What were the side effects associated with *z*? If *a* happened, would *b* take care of it? She seemed curious—every bit of information got a "Why?" But it wasn't curiosity as much as skepticism. Bob's illness required complicated treatment that carried a lot of risk and she wanted to know how much, and could we fix whatever might go wrong.

The answer to that was, no. No, we could not fix all the possible problems that might result from his stem cell transplant. No. Not even close.

I think he did have hard times during treatment. One day he showed me a poem he had written. An accountant, he worked from the hospital when he was able, and he'd written the poem on a single long, yellow sheet of paper from a legal pad. In the poem he saw himself as a lone wolf, abandoned and afraid. I wish I could remember it, wish I had a copy of it. The contrast between the friendly, unflappable Bob we always saw and the Bob who wrote that poem stunned me.

Here's the kicker. He didn't make it. There were too many complications from the transplant. Bob's obituary, in testament to Wendy, read (in paraphrase), "He is survived by his loving wife and champion of twenty-five years, who was his best friend and most excellent caregiver." That describes her; it really does.

I still don't know what about them made me reach for magic. I'd never felt that way before and haven't since, even though I've cared for lots of very ill and deserving people. I tend to be firm about the truth, advocating that everybody face the risks of medical care head-on, because that is the nature of informed consent to difficult treatment. But with Bob and Wendy, I only wanted to make his health issues go away. And that is why I wished, this one time only, to be a fairy godmother, a genie, maybe even a lesser god. I wanted a magic wand that worked and I wanted it to cure him.

But she was the one, I think, who drew me in, not him. Or it was them as a couple. Her questioning, her openness and spunk. If I'm honest, she struck me as a best-possible version of myself. And he, with his surface calm, his friendliness, in some ways reminded me of my husband. But I don't think I wished for magic because I thought no one like me should suffer, or that wanting to save them made me personally feel safer.

I think, instead, that because I identified with them, I could more readily imagine their pain. What, then, is the nature of compassion? Patients do not have to look like me or remind me of myself for me to care about them. And yet. When lives are at stake, compassion may become personal in a way that ideally it would not. I strived to treat all patients with identical solicitude and care, but how I *felt* about them was not always the same. Not only Bob and Wendy, but others, for varied reasons—a white mom with a PhD who also had three kids, a young Black man with a killer smile and the same initials as my husband, middle-aged wives worn to the nub by their husband's care and their doctors' failure to tell them the truth—those pulled harder at my heart.

I read *Cod*, the book I believe Bob had been reading. A few tidbits: the selling of dried, salted cod made the American colonies economically independent from Great Britain, setting the stage for the Revolutionary War. Cheap cod from America became the primary food of enslaved Africans on Caribbean sugar plantations, which meant the fish was essential to the slave trade. And overfishing of cod along the Newfoundland and New England coasts offers a cautionary tale about the importance of conservation. Something as ordinary as cod was part of all that history, and more.

Something else ordinary—a genetic mutation—can tell a cell to never stop dividing, and become a cancer. The thing about a cancer story, unlike a fish story, is that it's about a person. One person's history can change forever, or end, because of cancer. The survival rate on my floor of the hospital could go as low as 30 percent. Succeeding in this work requires seeing the good we do over time. There is too much sadness to feel every shift. Walls are necessary. But sometimes I touched the edges of my patients' hurt; it came so very close.

FOUR

First You Cry

HOME. I WANTED to go home after the scan. They told me not to drive myself, so I texted my twin daughters, Miranda and Sophia, newly moved into a nearby freshman dorm because they had started college a few weeks before. "I'm not feeling so good. Can one of you drive me?" It wasn't the full truth, but close enough.

Going against the radiologist's advice, I drove to their dorm, just ten blocks away, intending for one of them to take over when I got there. They could have walked to where I was, but I didn't want to admit I needed that. *Anyone can drive ten blocks*, I insisted to myself. However, between me and their dorm was a short street that connected the two main roads, Fifth Avenue and Forbes, that bisect the University of Pittsburgh campus. That short road, called Bigelow, was the only way for me to get to Miranda and Sophia's dorm, and three crosswalks bisected that block of Bigelow, including one on each corner and one in the middle of the street. During breaks between classes, many students used the middle crosswalk to cross the connecting road in large, amoebalike groups, which turned driving into a crawl, if that.

Classes must have let out right before I got on the connecting road, because many many students were using the crosswalk in the middle of the street. It was a horde of students, all oblivious to my bad news, and for the first time I understood, truly understood, why the sick sometimes envy the well. For them, it was an ordinary day, and I supposed, although perhaps wrongly, that none of them had just learned they had cancer. None of them had to tell their children they had cancer. None of them had an out-of-town husband who had no idea they probably had cancer.

I wanted them to get out of my way, to make a lane for me. These students with their book bags, their all-absorbing phones. Their indifference felt like an insult as I sat there, moving inches, for several minutes that seemed like forever. Even now, years later, I am in that car, on that street, watching student after student go through the crosswalk, while I wait, unable to move, burdened by the worst news of my life.

Eventually, the number of students lessened and the cars moved. My daughters were waiting outside their dorm. On the way home we picked up their older brother, my son, who lived off campus. I don't remember texting him, but maybe I had. I don't remember going into our house when we finally arrived, or anything, really, except for sitting on the couch and telling them that I had breast cancer. Or rather, that the doctor was pretty sure I had breast cancer.

I don't remember how I said it or what words I used. I don't remember the looks on their faces, but I do remember that they were calm. Is that normal? My surgeon's nurse told me later, "You're calm, so they're calm." Is that true? Was I calm? I was controlled, but is that the same as calm? Real calm? I do not know.

"Do I have to wear pink now?" I asked them.

Three decisive "Nos!" answered.

"Well," I said, "I thought maybe when you were told you had breast cancer you automatically got an oversized pink sweat-shirt that you had to wear all the time." They laughed. "You know, they say get a wig that matches your real hair, but that's no fun! I want a wig of spiky red hair!"

"Yes, Mom!" and "Go, Mom!" This was my chorus. They cheered for me.

My husband was due home that evening and I told them I would not call him, that no one wants to get that kind of information while waiting in an airport, to stew over on the flight. Him finding out a few hours later would not change anything, and there was nothing he could do, anyway.

"Do you want us to get you chicken noodle soup?" one of them asked.

"Yes. Yes!" Chicken noodle soup from our local Chinese noodle shop. I don't remember if I gave them money, or if they just went. I don't remember if I encouraged them to get food for themselves: vegetable dumplings, or a pizza from the take-out place a few stores down.

I do remember this: they brought back the soup and three kinds of junky candy I like from the drugstore. There was a huge Twix bar, a bag of Swedish Fish, and, and, and . . . none of us remembers the third thing. I have no idea what it might have been, even though I know I enjoy whatever-it-was as an occasional guilty pleasure.

Their father, my husband, Arthur—he's a physics professor at U. Pitt—got home from his work trip and I told him my likely diagnosis. I have no memory of any of it. None. I don't remember my words or the look on his face. Did he cry? How did the kids respond? What is the sound of silence? The sound and fury signifying nothing? Are they the same sounds as telling your husband of twenty-three years that you have breast cancer when afterwards you can't remember one thing you said?

Well, I do recall one thing: At some point I told my family that I couldn't stop crying after being diagnosed. *First, You Cry*: The book by Betty Rollin, a television newscaster, about her diagnosis of breast cancer and subsequent mastectomy, was published in 1976. The movie version, starring Mary Tyler Moore, was released in 1978. In 1978, I was thirteen. The memory of that book, that movie from my adolescence came to me somehow. "The books are right," I said, near the end of the evening. First thing—I had cried.

I couldn't drive without becoming enraged, couldn't get my own dinner, couldn't even think, but I remembered that book.

First, you cry.

And then what?

Newsflash: Rollin is still alive. She was diagnosed with breast cancer in her remaining breast in 1984 and had another mastectomy, but she's written books, directed news programs, lived her life. Deaths from breast cancer have also declined a lot, by 35 percent, since 1975, the year of Rollin's initial diagnosis.

At the same time, the incidence of breast cancer—the number of cases overall—increased by 25 percent. A popular explanation for that increase is that breast cancer is now "overdiagnosed." That is, mammography catches many early-stage breast cancers, and some researchers have confidently asserted that a percentage of those cancers would never become problems. Women, they say, are overscreened and overtreated for breast cancers that would never threaten our health.

I was formerly on that bandwagon. But there's nothing quite like having a mass in one's own breast to make an abstract certainty about the harm of overscreening seem completely irrelevant, even wrong. Right now at least, no test exists for determining exactly which cancers are aggressive, troublesome mutations and which ones aren't. No one knows for sure, and there is no cure for metastatic breast cancer, which killed roughly forty thousand American women in 2017, the year I was diagnosed. So, first you cry.

And then what?

You give up; you give in. *Upside down.* You're standing with your head on the floor, your feet reaching to the ceiling. You joke about wearing pink sweatshirts and punk-rock wigs. The children bring you dinner. Your husband, whom you love, becomes a well-intentioned blur.

Betty Rollin is still alive. But for me, from this point on, normal was over.

FIVE

Storytelling

BEAR WITH ME.

For my English dissertation I wrote about what I called "storytelling," meaning the use of stories to create community, and especially to create community for people whose voices have not always been listened to. That could mean patients, and it did—one of my chapters focused on poet and activist Audre Lorde's autobiographical book, *The Cancer Journals*. A Black woman, after her own breast cancer diagnosis and mastectomy, Lorde lamented that the only prostheses available to her were pink and thus didn't match her skin color.

Leslie Marmon Silko's book *Storyteller* got me interested in the concept of storytelling. It's an unusual collection of short fiction and nonfiction, poems, Indigenous American legends, and photographs. It lacks a table of contents and is wider than it is tall so that it does not fit easily on a regular bookshelf; it sticks out. Maybe that's the point. Silko identifies as a member of the Laguna Pueblo tribe in New Mexico, but she also has Mexican and Anglo-American ancestors. Her work often explores the friction between Indigenous American and non-indigenous, or white, culture.

There's a piece in *Storyteller* called "Tony's Story." In it, an Indigenous American named Tony and his older friend, Leon, who is newly returned home after serving in the army, are repeatedly harassed by a cop who has a history of violence towards the people he calls "Indians": "I don't like smart guys, Indian. It's because of you bastards that I'm here. They thought there wouldn't be as many for me here. But I find them." When Tony and Leon are at a fair on the reservation, without any warning or reason, the cop punches Leon in the mouth, knocking out some of his teeth and bloodying his face. Leon talks afterwards about how the cop violated his, Leon's, "rights" and insists, "He can't do it again. We are just as good as them." Tony thinks to himself, "The guys who came back always talked like that," as if the rules and "rights" of the white American world would be fairly applied to Indigenous people, when usually they were not.

Tony sees the cop completely differently than Leon. To Tony, the cop is an evil spirit, a witch who dresses in black and wears reflective sunglasses to hide "its" eyes. Tony wants Leon to forget about the cop because "it" is dangerous: "I knew that the cop was something terrible, and even to speak about it risked bringing it close to all of us."

The story has a macabre ending that nevertheless brings good fortune to the tribe. Tony and Leon are riding in Leon's pickup truck and the cop chases them in a patrol car, pulls them over, and tells them to get out of Leon's truck. Then the cop, raising a billy club high over Leon's head, says, "I'm going to beat the shit out of you . . . I like to beat Indians with this." Tony had dreamed of the cop as a witch who pointed a long human bone at him, and to him the cop's club is that bone "painted brown to look like wood."

"The shot sounded far away and I couldn't remember aiming," Tony narrates. He shoots and kills the cop before the cop hits Leon with the wooden club. Then Tony insists that he and Leon burn the cop's body after putting it back inside the patrol car. Leon, terrified at what Tony has done, stands "pale and shaking." But as the cop's blood soaks into the dry ground in the same pattern in which Leon's blood soaked the ground when the cop hit him at the fair, suddenly "in the west, rain clouds were gathering." A terrible drought had plagued the pueblo, and the killing of the cop, the ceremonial watering of the dry ground with his blood, has ended it and rain is coming.

That's how the story ends. It's gruesome, but I was enthralled by the contrast between Leon and Tony, the way Leon had embraced the language of laws and rights during his army service, and how Tony understood the cop's racism towards Indigenous Americans as a primal force that could only be stopped by equally fundamental violence. As I read, I felt the dryness of the land in my mouth and on my skin, and I appreciated how Silko's writing transformed the cop, in Tony's eyes at least, into an evil thing—Tony calling the cop "it"—that must be killed for the good of the tribe.

There's a twist to this story, though. In 1952 on Good Friday, a state trooper named Nash Garcia was killed and burned in his patrol car on the Acoma Indian Reservation (Acoma Pueblo borders on Laguna Pueblo—the Acoma and Laguna were neighboring tribes). Two brothers, Willie and Gabriel Felipe, who were from Acoma Pueblo, were arrested for the crime, confessed, and in 1953 were sentenced to death. A psychiatrist who examined the Felipes after their conviction found that both of them exhibited high levels of psychosis. They, like Tony, believed they were chased by witches and that witchcraft was a problem they had to handle as individuals, rather than as part of the tribal community. The psychiatrist made it clear that the Felipes' beliefs were singular, atypical of the Acoma, and compromised their understanding of law and morality to the point that they were legally insane. Being declared criminally insane saved the brothers' lives—they received reduced sentences of life imprisonment, rather than being slated for execution.

To write "Tony's Story," Silko drew on her memories of what people she knew had said about Nash Garcia at the time of his killing. He hated Indigenous Americans and used his authority as a state trooper to assault them without repercussions. But what fascinates me is that Silko only became aware of the psychiatrist's report on the Felipes a few years *after* she wrote the story. She had invented Tony's spiritual beliefs, which we could label psychosis.

I am not superstitious, but I often heard Tony's words in my head when I started working in oncology: "I knew that the cop was something terrible, and even to speak about it risked bringing it close to all of us." I wondered if taking care of cancer patients meant I had given cancer entrée into my own life. By which I meant that I had invited it into my body. I worried that by taking up my family history of cancer as a professional mantle, instead of running away from it, I brought danger to myself.

Of course, that's ridiculous.

The ultrasound tech who held me in her arms when I got the tentative-but-pretty-sure breast cancer diagnosis, who told me, pointedly, "They can cure this," also told me, "Cancer is the devil." I knew what she meant. Malignant and evil are close synonyms. The radiologist said my mass "looks ugly," which is to say, vile and malevolent. That doesn't mean I brought it closer by fighting in the trenches against it. Cancer is not the devil, but biology gone wrong: apoptosis—normal programmed cell death—on the fritz.

Leslie Marmon Silko's retelling of the killing of Nash Garcia gave the members of Laguna Pueblo a culturally mean-ingful way to understand his racism and his murder. That is the storyteller's after-the-fact power. I wish my storytelling could give me power over my cancer right now, but alas, diagnosis and treatment are the tools for conquering cancer, not stories. I might bleed during surgery, but my blood will not soak into the ground and work a miracle. There are no evil spirits and I know no rituals of healing. My choice to become an oncology nurse did not give me this disease, but if only my words, my stories, could cure it.

SIX

An Ideal Patient

A BIOPSY IS simple in theory: take a sample of tissue to look at under a microscope in order to determine whether it is cancerous. The "sample" must come from the tumor itself and be big enough for a pathologist to determine whether or not it contains cancerous cells. Getting the sample can be complicated, because even though the amount of tissue needed is relatively small, a biopsy typically requires cutting out a piece of someone's body. It's not surgery but a procedure, and the cutting can make it difficult.

When I was sixteen and still in high school in Missouri, I had two breast lumps, or tumors, surgically removed, one after the other, both benign fibroid adenomas, what I wanted to believe I had this time. Both times, during an office visit, the surgeon used a needle to determine whether the lumps were cysts. He stuck a long, slender needle into each lump, which means into each of my breasts, but could not extract fluid. My memory is that it didn't hurt, or at least not that much, and he decided on surgery after the failed fluid extraction, which showed that the lumps were not cysts. Back then, they—whoever in medicine makes these decisions—thought that benign tumors could turn malignant, so a surgeon would remove them. We now know that fibroid adenomas are not precancerous and I've had doctors and nurses snicker when I tell these stories, as if to say, *How stupid they used to be.* But it wasn't that long ago.

For each surgery they put me under with a general anesthetic and it took me a lot longer than normal to wake up, but I was fine. The first time, a visiting friend brought me a single red rose in a small white vase. After the second surgery, my dad cut blooming iris from the garden, put the flowers into a large glass, and placed it on my dresser. An abundance of green leaves and purple and indigo blooms cheered me while I healed.

I don't remember if they gave me any kind of pain medicine, or what the pain felt like, but I remember that there was pain. Pain and stitches, which fascinated me. Amazing that someone can sew up a body same as a hem on a skirt. That was then. Now we have a proliferation of tools to make biopsies easier so that they are "less invasive," an oxymoron. There are degrees of invasion, but I'm not sure invasiveness, in this instance, can ever truly be "less."

After the "I see a mass" ultrasound, I needed two biopsies. The radiologist was most concerned about the ugly growth in my right breast, the one almost in my armpit that looked like a star on the imaging. There were also calcifications in a different part of the same breast and she wanted a sample from that spot, too. Calcifications are areas where calcium deposits have clustered, and usually they are benign, but sometimes they result from precancerous changes in the breast, or they can indicate breast cancer. I had a possibility of two different kinds of breast cancer in one breast, or the same cancer in two different places in the breast, or one breast cancer in one place.

The day of the biopsies, I thought I was back in my element. I was a patient, not a nurse, but because I'm a nurse I knew what sort of patient to be: passive, undemanding, easy to manage. I strove to be that patient, because in general, easier patients receive better care. I've told patients to "be the squeaky wheel," because in certain situations, speaking up will get a patient more attention, but in general the smooth wheel makes quality care more likely.

I hate to admit that's true, but it is. Imagine a job that requires working with another person. Now imagine that that person constantly complains, throws up barriers to getting the work done, and generally makes every process take longer than it would otherwise. That's annoying, but worse, it gums up the gears, slowing things down, and since everyone on the front line in health care is overscheduled, they want tests and procedures to go smoothly because other patients are always waiting. Even a very reasonable request for gentleness, or basic consideration, can come across to techs and clinicians as trouble in the form of lost time. I learned, from my preceptor Carrie P., that such a calculus is wrong, but the system doesn't readily adjust.

Be the easy patient. I could turn the system to my benefit because I was part of it. That's what I told myself, without understanding that being the easy patient also has a cost.

The following are necessary characteristics for care to feel compassionate, according to Boston's Schwartz Center for Compassionate Healthcare: effective communication, emotional support, trust and respect, mutual decision-making, and treating patients as people, not just illnesses. None of that is easy. Easy is moving widgets along an assembly line. "Medical care without compassion cannot be truly patient-centered," insists Beth Lown, Chief Medical Officer at the Schwartz Center. She's right. Or as Hannah B. Wild, a Stanford medical student, affirmed in *Health Affairs* magazine, "Pain wants authenticity." A health care system focused on efficiency to protect revenue, rather than limit pain, doesn't put the patient at the center or allow much time for genuineness.

Two biopsies, back to back, meant double the pressure for efficiency. First, I would have what's called a stereotactic biopsy, to sample tissue from the area with the calcifications, and then a needle biopsy would take tissue from the mass on the far right side of my right breast. A stereotactic biopsy is one of the odder procedures in modern medicine—I knew this already because I'd had one before, in my early thirties, for a different set of noncancerous calcifications. The patient lies on a table with the selected breast dangling down through a hole in the table. Once the patient is in position, the table is elevated, making the patient feel like a car on a lift in a garage. The doctor works under the table, using X-ray imaging to localize the spot in the breast from which she needs a sample. The one thing they tell patients: don't move unless we ask you to.

My stereotactic biopsy took a long time, much longer than usual, I was told, because they couldn't zero in on the right spot. I lay on my right side, making, when they asked, micro-adjustments to my position. As my breast dangled through the hole in the table, my discomfort from lying in such an unusual position for such a long time turned into pain. At one point they took a break to let me stretch. Turning to look behind me, I saw three radiologists standing in what appeared to be the biopsy control center, pointing at a screen. I wondered if they were discussing how to get the correct angle. Three MDs, coincidentally all women, which comforted me, though I couldn't say why. Probably some sexist-derived hope that female physicians are kinder than male doctors. And why three MDs? I took it as bad news/good news: they couldn't get the sample they wanted, but they were working together and trying hard.

Really, though, I have no idea why three physicians were there. Throughout, the docs and techs told me little of what was happening. Removing tissue stings, but no one warned me before they did it. However, I felt reassured when I saw those three doctors conferring, their foreheads identically wrinkled in concentration. They were taking the crucial part of the biopsy very seriously, and afterwards they praised me for how calm I had been, how patient. It's pathetic to admit how much I appreciated that. During the test they forgot about Theresa the person, and I didn't complain, didn't ask for explanations, didn't move unless told to do so. I had turned myself into a body without a will. I did that to let them pay attention to their work, but someone there could have told me what was happening. The doctors focused on my right breast but, not to put too fine a point on it, that breast was attached to a human being and they knew that, even if the way the procedure was set up made it easy to forget.

The needle biopsy was more of the same. It took place in a different room with an ordinary, nonmovable table and I lay face up, with a triangular cloth-covered bolster stuck under my right side, elevating it. The team was again all women, including a senior radiologist and a fellow, a radiologist in the final stage of training. In this new setting, having women look after me did not feel comforting. On some level, which perhaps shows my age, I did enjoy watching female physicians use the hi-tech apparatuses of modern health care, focused not on me but on their work. It looked like progress of a sort: women displaying expertise without the expectation that they would be personable or kind. They weren't unkind, but they were impersonal and impersonal was hard to take. Pain wants authenticity.

The senior radiologist took a moment to explain to the fellow which tool she preferred for needle biopsies. The one the fellow most liked was not there. "Too expensive," the senior doc said, recommending a different one for the fellow to use. The instrument they ultimately chose looked like an overly complex staple gun. The techs positioned me carefully, propping me up with the bolster, placing my right arm just so, and again told me not to move. The mass being so close to the chest wall made the sample hard to get. As the fellow came near to me with her elaborate staple gun of a tool, she seemed to recognize the whole human being lying on the table in front of her. "I'm sorry," she said, "I'm so sorry." I wondered what she was apologizing for—the cancer, the biopsy, or both?

Modern health care is an assembly line. Procedures get done, codes get entered into computer systems, and money changes hands. Understanding how people feel about their illness, about their care, earns revenue for no one. You can't bill for empathy. It has no ICD-10 diagnosis code. I feel I should be thankful for that "I'm sorry" from the fellow, should be glad of it. But I'm not. *Just get on with it*, I wanted to say, tired of reclining at odd angles in dark rooms, my breasts exposed to strangers. The fellow's recognition of a whole person lying on the table came too late.

But when the biopsy was done, and they all congratulated me again on my "superhuman" patience, my stringent adherence to the passivity requirement, a tech held my hairband up to me. Made of a subtly zebra-patterned cloth with over-stretched elastic inside, the band never stayed put. It had slipped off during all the repositioning. "You don't want to forget your hairband," she said, holding it out balanced on her first two fingers. My heart filled with joy. Really—I felt joy. Because, to the tech at least, I was more than just a breast, coincidentally attached to a woman.

Researchers and physicians who assert that women are overdiagnosed for breast cancer say that they want to spare women "anxiety" from over-treatment. That sounds to me like paternalism, but their intentions are probably good. The standard treatment for breast cancer, beginning in 1882, was the disfiguring "radical mastectomy." Then in the early 1970s, Bernard Fisher, a surgeon, proved that lumpectomy plus radiation gave women the same chance of survival as mastectomy. Standards change, based on science, observation, and in the case of Fisher's lumpectomy recommendation, compassion for patients.

It is true that being diagnosed with cancer provokes anxiety, as does cancer treatment. Breast cancer specialists who are concerned about patients' anxiety could, instead of advocating for less screening and treatment, work to ensure that all women diagnosed with breast cancer receive humane care. They could pursue this important goal for all cancer patients, in fact, and even for seriously ill patients who don't have cancer. Being sick makes people anxious, but careful explanations, maybe a hand to hold while lying topless on a table, the giving back of a zebra-striped headband, can be healing, as they alleviate anxiety, too.

SEVEN

What We Talk About
When We Talk About Amputation

THIS IS A short story. It has two parts.

FIRST. THE PATIENT in the bed was an older woman. She was very large, meaning she was obese, and diabetic. I'm not sure why she had a bed on the medical oncology floor. She must have been moved from a more general floor that was full. She had diabetic ulcers on both her lower legs, and they were wrapped in thick dressings that looked like ACE bandages. The nightshift nurse told me we were to leave the dressings in place. And I did.

The next day, my next shift, I took care of the patient again. This was when I still worked in my first hospital job, with the bullies. As the morning wore on, I found myself being criticized by a few of the other nurses. They—or rather someone who, beneficently or not, clued me in—were saying behind my back that the dressings on the patient's legs needed to be changed daily and I hadn't changed them.

By this time the floor had a new manager, one without prior connections to the bullying nurses, one who didn't view naked aggression as normal for nurses on the floor. I stepped up to her office door to ask about the complaint. What should I have done? I didn't see an order for daily changes of the patient's bandages. If another nurse knew something about the patient that I didn't, she hadn't offered up that information.

I myself had no idea how to even begin with the patient's wounds. In nursing school I had learned the basics of wound care, but not wounds like these. Changing dressings on diabetic ulcers is not like taking off a peeling Band-Aid and replacing it with a new one. The wounds would need to be cleaned, have a healing agent applied, be covered with a specific type of bandage or gauze, and then rewrapped with thick dressings similar to what they were already wrapped with. Care of wounds involves so much technical knowledge that special wound care nurses often are called in to decide on the best treatment. In other words, the correct way to care for complex wounds must be learned. Medical oncology patients don't often have serious wounds, so it's possible that no nurse on the floor really knew how to care for this poor patient's legs. Maybe that's why they accused me of doing it badly.

Afraid that the new manager, whom I'll call N, had already heard about my failings with this patient and doubted my abilities, I simply told her that some of the nurses were saying I hadn't done my job with the patient's leg wounds. She looked at me with wide-open eyes. "I haven't heard that," she said.

For me, that was the end of it. If I had really screwed up, someone would have eagerly told N all about it. Indeed, no physician called me on the carpet, and neither did the patient or her family. Had there been an earlier order to change the dressings and no one wanted to do it? Or no one knew how? Carrie P., again Carrie P., always said, "This is a twenty-four-hour job." If I had neglected a task, the nurse following me should have done it, and then told me the next day, making sure I understood.

A study done in 2014 found that 17 percent of nurses leave their first job within a year, and a third leave within two years. A 2018 study found that half of all nurses had considered leaving nursing altogether over the prior two years and research shows that bullying contributes to burnout and to nurses quitting. I thought about quitting, thought I had misjudged my new field. But then I decided I had worked too hard to give up so quickly.

I also learned, months later, after I moved to the ward across the hall, that hospitals know when they have bad actors. Management knew about the problems on the floor, same as administrators know which doctors yell at staff and throw things. None of this is secret, even though similar behaviors in many other workplaces would lead to interventions, if not getting fired outright. Why did management not act? I don't know.

SECOND. THE PATIENT who may or may not have needed her dressings changed daily was scheduled for a below-the-knee amputation of both legs: a BKA. That's how bad her wounds were. The second day I took care of her, I prepared her as much as I could. Mostly I waited, as she did, too, because the operating room kept pushing back the time of her surgery. I had three other patients that day, and she didn't require much care from me, so I would look after my other patients, go back to her, and discover that the surgery had once again been delayed.

I was still a new nurse and didn't know that I could call the OR scheduler and ask what was up with all the postponements. Losing both one's legs below the knee is, well, traumatic, to say the least. The patient would never walk on her own two legs again. For her, the surgery was a huge deal.

Finally, word came. The operation would be tomorrow.

Tomorrow was a day too late. I spoke with the patient's son and daughter, adults who had taken time off work, rearranged their schedules, based on the fact that their mother would come out of life-changing surgery that day, not tomorrow. They were put out, especially since the OR didn't give a reason for postponing. No one, except for me, even said they were sorry to the patient.

The patient was Black, and Black Americans are often victimized by similar kinds of health care slights. Multiple examples of systemic racial bias in health care have come to light over the past few years, and if postponing the surgery resulted from discrimination, it reflects the racism extant in U.S. health care. One surprising example of such racism was recently discovered in commonly used algorithms of care. Multiple medical centers and federal health care agencies use computer algorithms to tag patients with challenging health issues who would benefit from intense personalized primary care. The objective is to give those patients regular care to keep them from needing highly expensive, catastrophic care. A standard algorithm puts patients into the highest risk group based on their health care spending, using money as a correlate for actual health care used. The problem with using money spent as a proxy for care received, as Ziad Obermeyer et al. wrote in *Science* when exploring this problem, is that Black Americans spend less on health care than white Americans, even when Black Americans have a much greater "disease burden" than whites.

Black Americans who are very sick tend to get less health care than comparatively healthier white Americans for many reasons, including that they cannot skip work to see a doctor, or afford the required co-pays, or get transportation to and from the clinic. "There are many opportunities for a wedge to creep in between needing health care and receiving health care—and crucially, we find that wedge to be correlated with race," the authors assert. The algorithm excluded Black Americans who would have benefited the most from intense primary care because the algorithm responded to their spending rather than their actual level of need.

I like that word *wedge*, because it felt like the patient had been wedged out of the OR schedule. I also wondered if a wedge—whether economic, situational, or personal—had kept her from receiving the diabetes care she needed to prevent a BKA. Her legs, abandoned by the health care system, were now to become wedges, remnants of their formerly whole selves. I don't know if racism was at work here; I don't know if the patient's race would have been obvious in the electronic medical record. The amputation could have been delayed due to an entirely different ingrained problem: rigid scheduling demands and thoughtlessness around others' suffering.

I saw the surgical intern—a first-year doc—who had been assigned to the case sitting at the nurse's station, working on the computer. Feelings about racism and indifference swirled in my head. I walked up to him and said something sharp about how could her surgery be postponed just like that, with no explanation as to why.

He didn't say much in response, but after we'd finished talking and I headed back down the hall, out of the corner of my eye I saw him stand up, swing around to face the intern sitting next to him and declare, with vehemence, "Don't they know I didn't want to push that surgery off to tomorrow?"

I felt suddenly so sad. It's known that medical students' level of empathy declines during the four years they spend in medical school. Some research disagrees, but doctors-in-training describe the effect as undeniable. This intern cared and I had assumed he didn't and essentially blamed him for what was not his fault, i.e. delaying the surgery. What goes around comes around. I am also imperfect. Because I had been subjected to unfair criticism and whispered condemnations regarding the care of this patient, I had imagined myself the only righteous person in the bunch. I didn't know how the intern felt about the patient's surgery being postponed. I didn't know how much he also cared. He didn't tell me; I didn't ask. And in that silence, a wound—no easier to treat or dress than the ones slowly destroying the patient's legs.

EIGHT

My Radiologist

THE RADIOLOGIST IN charge during my second biopsy made it clear that she did not give out results. She took tissue samples. Full stop. A pathologist would determine whether the cells were cancerous and then someone, I didn't know who, would confirm the diagnosis, or not, with me.

After the biopsy finished, I tried to ask about findings and she interrupted me, "We don't know any results." *But can't you tell from looking?* I wanted to ask. It seemed that cancerous tissue would be such a terrible deviation from normal that it had to be visible to the naked eye; that this doctor could look at the sample of tissue and *know.* Because *I* wanted to know.

But she didn't know, wouldn't know.

It was then that the tech gave me my hairband: "You don't want to forget your hairband." No, I didn't, and I didn't, thanks to her. Thanks to her, I left the biopsy room with my zebra-print hairband, briefly high on the tech's unexpected kindness.

I still didn't know whether I definitively had cancer, though, and went to check out with the nurse who had checked me in, in her small, windowless room. I had not liked her because she was aggressively cheerful. Being the easy patient felt like enough—I would not also ask myself to make small talk about the weather with staff. I returned to the nurse's office after the biopsies, only wanting to know my results or when I could expect to know them. The nurse might have told me when the pathologist's report would be ready. Instead, she told me what would make it *unlikely* for me to get the results anytime in the next two days. It was Wednesday, and she said that if she didn't hear from the pathologist by Friday at two p.m., I would not get a call from her telling me whether I had cancer until the next Monday morning.

I felt my field of vision contracting, felt the adrenaline, felt like I couldn't breathe. Did she understand what she was asking of me? When I said I wanted the results by Friday, she explained, "Well, you don't want to rush the pathologist, do you? They have to stain the cells and you want them to do that right."

"I'm a nurse," I said, "I know what pathologists do."

In the waiting room I told Arthur that the nurse had said I might not receive the biopsy results until Monday. We turned to leave and then I stopped. I tried to lift my feet to walk, but they wouldn't go. Four full days separated that Wednesday from the following Monday.

I went back to ask the receptionist about the results again, hoping that I had misunderstood. They wouldn't really make someone wait a whole weekend on a cancer diagnosis because of paperwork, right?

I tried to explain my problem to the receptionist, tried to be coherent, but my memory is that I spoke in a word salad of "results, biopsy, Monday, paperwork, diagnosis, nurse, and don't understand." No one wants to handle fuming patients if they can avoid it. The receptionist called the nurse and invited Arthur and me to come back through the office door and stand in the hallway. The nurse walked up to us and started with, "I already explained to you . . ."

I could narrate the entire conversation, but I won't. The biopsy would reveal whether I definitely had cancer, either setting me on a treatment path or giving me the biggest relief of my life. She had to know that. "We get the results in batches," the nurse said, "and I can only call you with a result once my radiologist has examined the results and signed off on them." She kept saying that: "*my* radiologist." *My* radiologist—hers, not mine. So, the pathologist told the diagnosis to the radiologist who performed the biopsy, and that radiologist told the nurse, who told me. But why was a phone call after two p.m. on Friday impossible? I asked if I could call the radiologist. "No!"

"You're telling me I might have to wait an entire weekend to find out if I have a disease that can kill me because of paperwork that's sitting on someone else's desk?"

And she said, "Well, I leave at four." So similar to that previous receptionist, who left the day of my diagnostic ultrasound without scheduling my biopsy, because even though her shift ended at three and I got to her desk at three, she was already gone. She must have finished her shift at 2:59, or earlier.

I know I was being demanding, and I support people leaving work on time, but a cancer diagnosis is something else: This nurse told me she leaves at four. Let that sink in.

Arthur and I left, but the nurse had given me a list of useful phone numbers, one of which was for making a complaint. In the car, going home after the test, while Arthur drove, I left possibly the most eloquent and outraged phone message of my life. I derided their focus on process. I used the word *cruel*. I knew what to say because I worked in that world, and I knew how to say it because I'm good with words. Through my job I'd learned to use the phone to get what I wanted for patients. That day *I* was the patient, and I used carefully worded rage to get what I wanted for myself.

It worked. After I got home, I called my internist, Dr. P and explained the situation. The next day—*the next day*—he called me and said that my complaints had made a difference. Then he gave me the results: "Yes, you have breast cancer," on the right side of my breast and not amid the calcifications. I am thankful that Dr. P recognized that I badly needed this news.

I realized, after I left the building where I had the test, that the nurse did not know that the initial radiologist, the one who did the first ultrasound, had told me she "saw a mass." That doctor, who afterwards spoke to me so gently in the dark room where she worked, was 99 percent sure I had cancer. I guess the nurse saw me as one more woman there for a screening biopsy that would in the end reveal nothing of concern. Or maybe she just didn't care. I can't rule that out.

Because the next day, when I knew my results were in the computer and available, she never called to tell me that I had cancer. Nor the day after, nor even the following Monday.

That nurse never called me.

Let that sink in, too.

NINE

Reason Not the Need

IT WAS THE Fourth of July and I was working at my first nursing job, on the difficult floor. The day before I had worked 7 a.m. to 3 p.m. and then 7 p.m. to 11 p.m: it was the coverage they needed. I agreed, knowing I had to be in at 7 a.m. the next day, a holiday. But as a reward, the charge nurse shortened my July Fourth shift from twelve hours to eight. I would leave the hospital at 3:30 p.m., not four hours later, free to celebrate the holiday with Arthur and the kids.

The odd hours left me pretty tired and that morning, before I got to work, I ordered a large iced latte with an extra shot of espresso at the coffeeshop across the street from the hospital. I hoped the extra shot would wake me up. Not much happens in hospitals on holidays. The docs do their rounds quickly and sometimes a new attending will sub for the usual person. This one-day physician defers all but the simplest decisions, not wanting to upset the apple cart, which means not wanting the usual doctor to get upset with them for changing the treatment plan. The day becomes a placeholder, mostly, which drives patients crazy, but that's how it is. Anyone who can take the day off does.

Except for one of the oncology surgeons on that particular holiday. One of this doctor's patients was well enough to go home, but she needed her implanted port removed first. I thought that had to happen in an operating room, but I guess the ORs weren't open for such trivialities on the Fourth of July, so the surgeon opted to do the procedure at the bedside. I asked the charge nurse if that was OK. She stared at me for a minute and then slowly said, "Yes, sometimes they do that," an answer I found inscrutable but also understood was not "no."

A port is a quarter-sized appliance about one-fourth of an inch thick that gets surgically implanted under the skin of a patient's upper chest. It has an attached tube that feeds into a central vein going into the heart. When a port needle is inserted through the skin, into the port, intravenous drugs that need to go through what we call a central line are infused through the port via the attached tube. It's kind of a genius invention, since most central lines have tubes for attaching IVs that protrude from the patient's chest or upper arm. With a port, patients can shower, swim, take baths, without worrying about keeping their IV line dry (to prevent infection).

For whatever reason, this woman's—my patient's—port needed to come out and the surgeon, whom I'll call Dr. C, planned to remove it in her room, that day. Dr. C had arranged for a set of surgical tools to be available to him on our floor, but when I called the OR asking when the tools would be delivered, they said, oh no, the tools wouldn't be delivered. I needed to pick them up. I was tired and amped-up on caffeine, banking on that extra shot to take me all the way through to mid-afternoon, when I would leave. Pick the tools up? Er, OK.

Remember—holidays, in general, are not busy. I had time to go to the OR holding area and get the collection of tools, or rather, pick up a heavy metal container that was roughly about two-and-a-half feet long, one foot wide, and one foot deep. I got off the elevator on our floor and lumbered down the hallway with the heavy box. An aide asked, wide-eyed, what I was doing.

I don't really know what I was doing. I guess I was doing my job. I had never met Dr. C before, but it was clear he played by his own rules. Well, that was fine. I wasn't that busy, so anything for the patient.

Dr. C was very friendly with the patient and talked with her as if he knew her and cared about her. I liked that. He was quick, too. He took out the port and sewed up the incision faster than I would have thought possible. He used maybe three items from the heavy container, which I now had to carry back down the hall, onto the elevator, and into the OR waiting room. I was mentally preparing myself to lift and return the toolbox as Dr. C walked down the hall to where we kept the charts, ready to put in discharge orders for the patient, then abruptly turned around and hurried back to me. "We forgot something," he said.

Hmmmm. *We? What is this "we,"* I wondered.

There's an old joke about the Lone Ranger, that masked hero of TV Westerns, and Tonto, his Indigenous American partner.

They are on horseback, trapped in a canyon, and surrounded by Indigenous Americans who seem threatening. The Lone Ranger turns to Tonto and says, "What are we going to do?" And Tonto replies, "What do you mean, 'we,' white man?"

Turns out "we" forgot to consent the patient. Good thing it was a holiday, when all the rules were a little bit off and Dr. C had already decided to go rogue. "We" consented the patient—had her sign forms agreeing to the surgery—after the fact. She didn't mind at all; whatever it took to get her out of the hospital was just fine with her.

Feeling half like a hero and half like a fool, I carried that heavy metal surgical box back to the staff in the OR. No one said anything to me, and I have never seen a nurse, or anyone else, carry one of those boxes around the hospital prior to that day or at any time after.

IT'S NOW TIME for some Shakespeare. *King Lear* has a resonant and oft-quoted line that's relevant here: reason not the need. It means we all have irrational desires, things we want, but can't say we need. Food, shelter, and clothing are considered essential needs for humans, but beyond those necessities, humans want many other things: companionship, interesting work, respect, love.

Lear has to defend his nonessential needs because he chose to relinquish his crown, giving authority over his kingdom to two of his three daughters. In case anyone is wondering, this is not a good idea. One either is or is not a king and monarchy cannot be separated from responsibility and authority, especially at the time *King Lear* is supposed to have taken place. But Lear divided his kingdom, giving his daughters the authority and power he once had. He expected gratitude and accommodation befitting, well, a king, in return. His intention was to live with both his daughters, alternating visits between their households. Lear's Fool, his wise court jester, believes Lear has made a mistake in setting up his daughters to rule over him, and tells him so: "Thou hadst little wit in thy bald crown when thou gav'st thy golden one away." Lear painfully learns to regret his decision only when he realizes his daughters will not house him in the manner he feels entitled to, and ultimately will not house him at all.

Because Lear had been a king, his wants were majestic in size. He expected a retinue of fifty knights on horseback to accompany him wherever he stayed. The scene where Lear's daughters completely disabuse him of this notion is spare and brutal. His daughter Goneril ticks down the number of knights Lear actually "needs" since her own servants are sufficient for the task of supplying his wants:

> Hear me, my lord.
> What need you five-and-twenty, ten, or five
> To follow in a house where twice so many
> Have a command to tend you?

Daughter Regan rhetorically slips in the knife immediately after, insisting that Lear does not need any retainers when he visits. "What needs one?" she asks.

Then Lear cries out:

> *O, reason not the need! Our basest beggars*
> *Are in the poorest thing superfluous.*
> *Allow not nature more than nature needs,*
> *Man's life's is cheap as beast's.*

Even beggars have *something* beyond the essentials, Lear implies, a little more than "the poorest thing." If Lear only receives what he deserves according to what "nature needs," he is being treated no differently than an animal.

There is another side to this story, maybe. Lear's men were uncouth, rude to members of his daughters' households, and unruly. Which of us, even if we lived in a castle staffed by servants, would want a visitor who brought fifty people with him? So maybe the daughters are not so unreasonable, except that the play does not unfold that way. Lear was a difficult and demanding father, but Goneril and Regan are exposed as villainous as the play proceeds. They are unkind, yes, but also greedy and violent. Their argument over how many retainers Lear truly needs ends with him being shut out of the castle and mostly left to fend for himself in a terrible storm.

REASON NOT THE need for a port to be removed at the bedside on the Fourth of July and for the nurse to carry an unwieldy box of surgical tools to and from the patient's room to make that port removal possible. Reason not my willingness to appear foolish, because I know I did. The day before, when I said I would end my shift at 3 p.m., return to the hospital from

7 to 11 p.m., then come back the next morning at 7 a.m., one nurse called my decision "stupid" to my face.

But that stupid choice let me leave early on July Fourth, which made watching fireworks with the kids and Arthur in downtown Pittsburgh possible. Fireworks are magical—the explosions of color, fantastic patterns, and showers of sparks and light. If I had to do it all over again, when Dr. C said "we" had forgotten something I might have, with the benefit of experience, cocked my head to one side and asked, "'We,' Dr. C?" Otherwise, I'd agree to work the same odd hours and lug that heavy box around the hospital. I wouldn't reason the need. For no one can say they *need* fireworks, or a holiday with their husband and children, but like Lear, we all at times want our "superfluous joys" satisfied.

TEN

Revelations

AFTER A CANCER diagnosis comes the necessity of telling people. Parents, friends. How would I do that? The C-word brings a weird aura into the conversation; it's part of the fear. You can hint around, say you have bad news, ask the person you're trying to tell if they "have a minute," maybe even make sure they are sitting down, but that's so clichéd I don't know if anyone actually does it. All that is avoidance of what no one ever wants to say: "I have cancer."

I started with my mother, who lives in Chicago. I called her and I told her. She drew in her breath and said "What?" as if she heard me wrong, as if the wrong words had come out of my mouth. Then something unexpected happened. She asked how long I had known and I told her about the mammogram, the follow-up, the biopsy, waiting for the official, pathologist-confirmed diagnosis of breast cancer. I said I didn't want to tell her until I was sure because I knew it would be hard not to know for sure. I am her only daughter.

But I didn't really spare her, because she had felt a distance between us over the past several weeks. She had worried that she had somehow offended me and had written me a letter asking if something was wrong. After hearing my news, she told me to throw away the letter, which I did, without reading it, when I received it a few days later.

I asked her to tell my brother and his wife, and his ex-wife, who remains a friend. They all live in Chicago and I asked her to take that burden from me, but I didn't say it like that. I mumbled something like "Can you tell them?" I didn't say why. I didn't say that telling her had been so painful and I imagined that telling my brother would feel the same. All this because of my one-centimeter cancer.

My talk with my mom had been brief, but when I got off the phone, I was exhausted. I needed to tell my dad, but I simply could not do it that same day. I told him the next day instead. But before I get to that, I need to make clear that there is a lot of water under the bridge between me and my dad. OK, the truth? My parents divorced when I was ten. With my dad, there's been a lot of drinking, also affairs, plus three wives, my mom being the first, the second being not only an alcoholic but mentally ill: she once set her own hair on fire. That woman, who died over a decade ago from a brain tumor, was my stepmother for years. My dad's still alive so I won't belabor the point. Lots of things could have been better. I worked with what I had.

I do not call him that often. Weeks go by, sometimes months, between phone calls, and I never return to southwest Missouri, where I grew up. I just don't. But I called him the next day, as I'd planned, and told him about the cancer. And his reaction really stunned me. Like my mother, he breathed in, said "What?" as if he hadn't heard correctly, but I heard something else in his tone that went a long way towards closing up the rift between us: he was shocked and he was sorry.

He was terribly sorry. People who have always been able to trust their parents, who haven't had mentally ill stepmothers and drunken fathers to deal with, will likely not understand. But here it is—my dad saw me. He saw me. And that was a gift.

That doesn't make my cancer a gift. Cancer is never a gift and when people with cancer say it is a gift—yes, people with cancer say that—I don't understand what they mean. But that moment with my dad—that was the world's smallest silver lining. It was enough. One word: "What?" It was the way he said it. Pain, but also—from the Latin *solari*, meaning to console or comfort—solace.

ELEVEN

I Lost You

AFTER I LEFT the hospital where I got my I-see-a-mass breast cancer diagnosis, after I walked out without an appointment for a biopsy, after I met up with my daughters and son, and then went home and told my kids and my husband that I very likely had breast cancer . . . after all that, actually the next day, I called my supervisor in home hospice and asked her to call me back.

When she called back, the reception was terrible. I tried to interject "I," "breast cancer" and "probably" in between the dead spots. "Oh, Theresa, that's terrible," she said, and then I heard only static.

I said "I lost you" over and over, gripping the phone tightly. The call was failing and I wanted to say more, to tell her that I would be taking a leave. I knew that I could not be a hospice nurse and a cancer patient at the same time. I was afraid of dying. But I only heard pieces of words from her, split up by static. I hung up. At least I had tried, and though it didn't seem right to text my likely breast cancer diagnosis, that's what I did.

Maybe it will be easier to write this, I typed, telling her that my diagnosis had not yet been confirmed with a biopsy, but they were pretty sure based on the imaging. *I need to take a leave*, I continued. *I will let you know the results when I know.* I switched to home hospice from hospital nursing in part because I wanted to care for patients in a setting that was personal for them and their family members. Now I had become a patient, pulled into the impersonal environment of modern health care.

Once I learned the actual diagnosis, I didn't even try to call; I emailed her. I had a casual, or *per diem*, position, so I could quit abruptly, without leaving the other nurses too much in the lurch. It turned out to be easy to leave my job—both a relief and a disappointment. My entire hospice team met every other week and I went to the next team meeting to say good-bye. I thought I would cry, but I didn't. I talked to them mostly about all the things I no longer remembered now that I was the sick one, which included almost everything I had ever learned about breast cancer. "I don't like being on the other side," I told them. "I'm used to being the one in control." Everyone nodded. *Yes. We understand.*

"I will definitely be back." It was the last thing I said before leaving the meeting and I'm not sure why I said it. Maybe I wanted to imagine they would all be waiting for me, or maybe I briefly saw myself in the made-for-TV movie version of my life. There's generally no prevarication among hospice staff, no lying about illness and prognosis. My colleagues said good-bye, good luck. What else could they say? I was the one lying. I smiled, worked hard to look brave, when I wanted to crumple to the floor, cry out, "I don't want to die!" and, sadly, "I've failed you!" I'd tapped into the paradox that binds American health care workers: that despite taking care of very sick people every day, we tend to believe that we are invulnerable.

A couple months later, I met my supervisor for lunch to give her my equipment: laptop, power cord, car charger, phone, phone charger, portable document scanner, tubes for blood samples, catheter kits, enemas, wipes, gauze in different sizes, wound dressings, and tubes of MediHoney, close to a miracle cure for simple wounds. The sky was gray, which matched my mood, and my inability to find a parking spot nearby felt like an injustice. It was nice to see her, though, to enjoy a bit of work gossip and catch up. But I remember one thing she said: "You have to be afraid of it coming back." "It" of course being cancer. I'm not sure why she said it, but this manager could be socially clumsy. Still, when she said that, I froze. On the list of things she could have brought up, I would have put "risk of recurrence" at the very bottom. I dealt with that nagging fear of death every day; I didn't need to be reminded that cancers return, that a cancer diagnosis can feel like a life sentence even when the cancer is small and slow-growing.

Fear messes with your mind. I've known nurses and doctors who worked through their cancer treatment. I don't know why they were able to do it when I couldn't. Maybe they were less afraid than I was, or maybe they never acknowledged their fear, or maybe they had to work—I knew how lucky I was in that regard. Arthur and I could pay our bills without my nurse's salary, so I could rest during treatment. I made money from my writing and from giving talks, and combined with what Arthur earned as a professor, we had enough. For those cancer patients who have to work, because they won't be able to pay the rent otherwise, or because they can't take time off without losing their jobs, or because they lack health insurance and legitimately fear the costs of treatment will bankrupt them, I assert that the United States, the richest country in the world, could do better by them. I only know that I could not be a cancer patient and a hospice nurse at the same time. Do you know these lines from Ecclesiastes?

> *There is a time for everything,*
> *and a season for every activity under the heavens:*
> *a time to be born and a time to die . . .*
> *a time to keep and a time to throw away,*
> *a time to tear and a time to mend . . .*

A time to tear and a time to mend. It makes sense, but I had never applied that dichotomy to myself: A time to care for others and a time to be cared for? Maybe so. A time to work and a time to heal, for me, I guess. Of course. Regret about not working dogged me, though. Struggling to accept my vulnerability, I couldn't escape a feeling of failure.

I grew up with an ingrained sense that being unwell was shameful or psychosomatic, or both. My dad literally called physicians quacks, though now that he's older he goes to the doctor more or less when he needs to. That's what vulnerability can do—wise you up to the realities of human frailty. But we all know people who look at acknowledging sickness as akin to sin, right? The people who righteously say they never take pills, not even aspirin. The people who come to work with fevers and insist they are fine. A nurse on my floor once showed up for her shift knowing she had pink eye and would be sent home, but that way she didn't get blamed for a call-off, never mind that the rest of us worked short-staffed that day because it was too late to get a sub.

Friends of mine not in health care imagine that hospitals do not want health care workers to come in sick, but that's not true. It is quite common for nurses who are indisposed to be tacitly labeled malingerers, as if poor health really is all in our heads. A time for everything ideally would include being able to take off work when unwell without having to fret over losing the respect of one's peers, or worse, one's job. But there's no slack in the system, so administrators maintain adequate staffing by, it seems, belittling workers' health issues (the irony). Every Australian, on the other hand, gets four weeks of mandated paid sick leave. *Four weeks.* Their economy has not ground to a halt as a result. Americans' obsession with productivity, our national focus on work as a moral value, does not benefit the ailing or those who care for them.

PART TWO

Nurse Brown, MIA

TWELVE

Balance

THIS WAS THE moment of the seesaw. The balance tipped from nurse to patient. Remember seesaws? They've disappeared from playgrounds—probably too dangerous. But seesaws gave valuable lessons in cooperation and the temptations of raw power. The friend who got on the seesaw opposite me would push off the ground on her end, sending her up and me down, and I would in turn push myself up and off, letting her back down to the ground. It felt like synergy, easy and rhythmic. That same friend could become an enemy, though, by calling over another classmate and combining their weights to keep their end of the teeter-totter down on the ground, leaving me fixed, high up in the air, legs uselessly kicking. I could try different strategies to convince them to let me down: insist, get mad, laugh it off, pretend I loved hanging out five feet above the ground, but in truth I was stuck. If those kids were really mean they would release me by suddenly jumping up off their end of the seesaw, causing my end to crash down, banging my butt, making my legs jerk up, and forcing my teeth together so hard they hurt.

A cancer diagnosis is, in its own way, a seesaw. And maybe also a bully, the same as those kids on the playground.

One of the last patients I visited before being diagnosed with cancer myself was a woman on home hospice with breast cancer. She lived in one of Pittsburgh's historically Black low-income neighborhoods. The husband of one of our new nurses had supposedly forbade her from caring for patients in that neighborhood. "Forbade"—even without the sexism in the husband's pronouncement, the word sounds like an ancient prohibition.

In truth, Pittsburgh crime statistics do show a not insignificant rate of violent crime for that neighborhood—and the husband's attitude reflected an even larger societal problem of poverty being linked with crime—but the ideal in health care is we treat all comers and we treat them the same no matter where they live. That's one definition of compassion. In the U.S., though, we absolutely do not treat all patients the same. For example, inability to pay is a known limit on access to care, enforced by insurance companies and hospitals alike, and is also structurally supported as a hard stop on care availability, except for those poor enough to qualify for Medicaid, or those over sixty-five, who qualify for Medicare. Our nurse's husband may have been worried about his wife's safety, or he may have had racist ideas, or both, but the truth is, equal care is already denied many people of color—sometimes because they can't pay, yes, but sometimes only because they are not white.

Cancer treatment specifically is unequal for Black Americans.

According to the American Cancer Society, "Black people have the highest death rate and shortest survival of any racial/ethnic group for most cancers in the U.S." For breast cancer patients, the mortality rate for Black women is almost twice the rate for white women. Black singer Marian Anderson famously described the subtlety of racism as "Prejudice: Sometimes it's like a hair across your cheek. You can't see it, you can't find it with your fingers, but you keep brushing at it because the feel of it is irritating." In health care, it seems, that hair on the cheek is often accompanied by a slap across the face.

I had been this patient's nurse maybe a month before (*per diem* nurses never have a set patient list) and my hope is on that day, for that patient, the care I gave was the same care I would have given anyone else. The patient had moved into her daughter's small two-story house, and they'd put her hospital bed in the first-floor living room against a side wall, in front of the TV and a large picture window. A kitchenette in the back filled out the space. I remembered her because when I saw her one month previously, she had refused all pain medication despite obviously being in pain.

That first time, when I came to the house, the patient wouldn't meet my eye as I asked about her pain and said the medications we offered could help. Her daughter came down the stairs and hinted that I should keep the visit short. Later, standing on the porch outside, the daughter told me that her mother hated having nurses in the house and hated the idea of taking narcotics for pain. I don't remember what I said, something along the lines of, "If she could only try the long-acting narcotic . . ." This is how it goes sometimes. People have all kinds of reasons for not wanting to take opioids and they won't always explain, or can't.

When I checked in a month later, though, the patient was transformed. She sat up straight in the hospital bed and looked right at me. Her white hair was combed back from her smiling face and she told me she had no pain at all: a small miracle of persistence and persuasion. She had started taking the medication. The daughter wasn't there, which meant another goal had been accomplished: the daughter could leave the house to go to work. When I'd finished the visit, as I got ready to leave by putting my stethoscope, thermometer, and blood-pressure cuff into my bag, the patient told me, "I'm going to beat this. I've just got too much living to do." She looked out the window at the street outside, and then back at me. "I've got grandchildren, you know."

I paused. Another seesaw—truth versus denial. Was this why she now took pain medication? Did she believe that she would survive her untreatable metastatic breast cancer? Hospice work demands scrupulous honesty about life and death to avoid giving patients false hope, but this time, for once, I hedged, tacitly supporting her denial. "Well, why not?" I told her. Then I smiled and waved as I left the house. Why not.

Why not. This woman, dying of breast cancer, is the last work memory I have prior to my own diagnosis. The specialized knowledge that comes from working in health care can feel like power, *is* power when a patient doesn't comprehend the likely outcome but we do. And that's part of why none of us wants to be in the hospital bed instead of standing next to it in scrubs.

But figuratively I was in a hospital bed, having forgotten almost everything I knew about cancer when I was diagnosed. Staging? Tumor markers? What the presence or absence of different chemical receptors, including estrogen (ER) and human epidermal growth factor receptor 2 (HER2), mean for treatment and prognosis? ER+ and HER2–? It might as well have been written in Sanskrit. What I did remember is that people die from cancer and sometimes their deaths are horrible. That was my clinical reality—what my nursing taught me—from working with acute leukemia patients and stem cell transplant recipients. Breast cancer, even breast cancer that has spread, isn't usually horrible in the sense of gruesome, but the sickest cancer patients end up in the hospital. There was a selection effect for bad news.

I'd somehow gotten on the wrong side of the seesaw. My balance was off. And I didn't have acute leukemia or lymphoma. I had a small, slow-growing tumor that was very treatable due to being estrogen and progesterone positive (ER+/PR+) and HER2 negative (HER2–). However, that diminutive mass had made my mortality real. My wee tumor—not palpable to touch, only detected on a follow-up ultrasound—scared me to death.

Modern health care saved me, saved my life, but Theresa the person got lost. We discuss physical failure in health care in terms like decompensation, morbidity and mortality, multiple organ dysfunction syndrome, and the patient ceased to breathe. But what about the soul, or whatever one calls that singular essence that makes each of us who we are? That needs tending, too. All I wanted after my diagnosis was for someone involved in treating my cancer to sit down with me, look me in the eye, and explain my diagnosis, discuss what my prognosis looked like, and clarify my likely course of treatment. That's it. Simple. Easy. Never happened. Another fulcrum: the separation in health care of patient and person, body and soul.

My friend H, who's an oncology nurse practitioner; my friend O, who's a surgical oncologist; and my internist, Dr. P, did it in bits and pieces. But no one who should have done that, whose job required them to do that—whether the surgeon, medical oncologist, or a trained nurse navigator—did. No one. My treatment took place at a so-called cancer center, but no one there did anything to manage my fear or calm my soul by explaining the process. No one helped me make appointments. No one talked about how long treatment would likely take. No one—except for the ultrasound tech—told me, "We can treat this."

That is failure, and when I felt this failure, felt it hurting me over and over again, I knew that it was also *my* failure as a nurse. It is a failure of compassion, which is not surprising since over the past few decades, health care has changed from people-centered to profit-centered. Profit makers focus on revenue, not feelings. Diagnosis-related groups (DRGs) and the International Classification of Diseases, Tenth Revision (ICD-10) billing codes do not address a clinical lack of compassion, but slighting the human in patients and clinicians alike shows we've got the balance wrong.)

Can we try again? Why not. People failed me when I was a patient and I failed patients when working as a nurse. I see that now. People also came through for me, and as a nurse I did my best for patients. But the overall balance between profit and compassionate care is off; it has tipped too far towards profit, meaning the playground bullies control the seesaw. Consider that more than twenty-five million Americans lack health insurance. Medical mistakes are one of the leading causes of death in the United States. Life expectancy in the U.S. is going down, not up. America spends more money on health care than any other industrialized country and our outcomes overall are much worse. These data points show how little patient well-being matters relative to the money-hungry health care machine. We can try, though, to restore the balance, to find that synergy in the seesaw, by caring equally for all patients, by treating the body *and* the soul.

THIRTEEN

Bedside Manner

I PICKED MY surgeon based on the recommendation of my friend O, who's also a surgeon. I explained that I didn't want a friend to be my surgeon and asked him who should do my surgery instead. "I have three recommendations for you," he said, "Bob Smith, Bob Smith, and Bob Smith." The surgeon's name wasn't actually Bob Smith, but I'll call him Dr. S anyway. "He's quirky but brilliant," O told me.

I could do quirky. Brilliant sounded good, too. Later, after my lumpectomy, I learned that in Dr. S's younger years, quirky meant out of control. He sometimes threw things in the OR and regularly yelled at people, or so I was told. Before my surgery, though, I wasn't concerned about those negative stories. All I knew was that Dr. S would save me—a heavy load, but that was his job.

For my appointment, which I think O helped me get sooner than I might have, though he never said as much, Dr. S came into the small examining room with an entourage: him, the nurse who always worked with him, and a surgical fellow. I sat on the paper-covered exam table, the back raised up behind me to form a makeshift chair. Arthur sat in the corner in a straight-backed chair, holding his large workbag firmly on his lap with both arms, covering up his chest.

When Dr. S asked me how I knew O, I told him it was one of those work friendships that lasted. Then Dr. S started to talk about my diagnosis, stopped, and looked over at Arthur. "Who are you?" he asked.

"I'm her husband."

"Well, I don't know," Dr. S said, "You could be the bus driver." *What? The bus driver? Was he joking?*

Dr. S dove in. He drew a breast on the small whiteboard in the room. He threw out statistics about my recurrence risk, which was low. At one point he said, waving his hand dismissively, "Don't even worry about the cancer you have now. That's nothing. We're planning for the next one." Huh. That was not what I wanted to hear. *The next one?* He also said that if I had a BRCA1 or BRCA2 genetic mutation—the most problematic mutations for breast and ovarian cancer—then I should seriously consider having a double mastectomy. I countered that breast cancers from BRCA1 and 2 mutations were always very aggressive, and mine wasn't, or at least I had heard that. "No. That's not true," he said. "That's a misnomer."

Oh. I thought I had an ace up my sleeve. Because I didn't have an aggressive breast cancer *now*, I *couldn't* have a genetic predisposition to breast cancer, and therefore I *wouldn't* need to think about having a mastectomy. Risk, unfortunately, cannot be assessed that simply, at least not for me. Here's what complicated the question of a possible genetic mutation: since my mother's mother and three of my mother's sisters had breast cancer, that put me in a higher risk group for one or both of the genetic mutations that made developing an aggressive breast cancer, and possibly ovarian cancer, more likely. Risk assessment is a mathematical calculation with room for error, not an absolute, and my genetic status mattered because it would shape my treatment decisions. If I lacked the BRCA1 and 2 mutations, I would be a good candidate for a surgical lumpectomy plus radiation only—no mastectomy needed. My risk of having my present cancer return would also be low if I did not have a BRCA mutation. But if I had one or both of the BRCA mutations, Dr. S would encourage a double mastectomy, what he called "the full Angelina Jolie," because Angelina Jolie, the movie star, had a prophylactic, or preventive, double mastectomy and oophorectomy (removal of her ovaries) after learning she had both BRCA mutations. Jolie's mother died in 2007 of ovarian cancer.

Dr. S wanted me to have genetic testing to check for the mutations, but he'd asked me by talking in circles, and afterwards, I think I figured out why. A few years before, I had a screening interview with a genetic counselor to determine whether testing for the BRCA1 and 2 mutations made sense for me. Would looking for a genetic predisposition to breast cancer be helpful? Based on my family history of cancer, the genetic counselor concluded that genetic testing would not benefit me because my statistically tabulated risk of having one of the worst-case mutations came in just below the level at which screening was advised. After thinking over the counselor's advice, I decided to follow her recommendation to not be tested. However, my new breast cancer diagnosis, combined with my family history, landed me back in the high-risk group, once again making genetic testing a relevant question.

What I think happened with Dr. S was that my earlier choice not to be tested must have been recorded in my chart as "declined genetic testing," or worse, "refused genetic testing," because that's how we say things in health care. Patients "fail" chemo, not the other way around, when their cancer isn't cured by treatment. Patients who do not follow medical advice get labeled "noncompliant," no matter the reason for their behavior. And patients who decide against screening can be said to have "refused" it, even if, like me, they were following medical advice when doing so. That could be why Dr. S talked around and around the question of testing, instead of directly recommending it and seeing what I would say. I wondered if he felt like he had to persuade me, since I had "refused" screening a few years before.

But maybe the explanation is even simpler. After I agreed to genetic testing, Dr. S laid me back onto the table, preparatory to examining me, and said, "Here's the problem; results take three weeks." He held up three fingers for emphasis. *Three weeks.* It sounded like forever. He did the exam, helped me sit up again, and left without saying another word. *What a strange man,* I thought. I wondered if I had gotten "the full Dr. S," the quirky brilliance that O warned me about.

In the meantime, I would wait three weeks to find out if a lumpectomy would suffice, or if I needed a double mastectomy. Those three weeks ended up being only two, but it felt like forever. Time stretched painfully. The seconds, minutes, and hours of every day passed like the clock hands were stuck in molasses. I remember so little from those two weeks, except for two talks I gave. I lectured to a law school class in Pittsburgh on "Communication: The Achilles Heel of Health Care." I left Dr. S's office and gave that talk almost right after, the same day. I also traveled to DC to speak to a specialized medical organization. My subject was "Quality Patient Care: It Takes a Team." Something about that title now feels sadly ironic.

The genetic counselor called me a week early. She sounded so serious, but then she told me I was negative for every mutation they knew to test for. Every single mutation. I felt relieved and also that waiting one more second to get my results would have been too much to bear, that I would have exploded, imploded, or spontaneously combusted from mental strain. For two weeks, my mind had been a TV screen tuned to a station of static gray. Those five words, "You are negative for everything," lifted the gray and the multicolored richness of our world rushed back in. I still had breast cancer, but I did not carry the genetic version of a family curse: I could not pass a genetic tendency for breast cancer down to my two daughters. I would not need to have both breasts surgically removed to save my own life.

The next and last time I saw Dr. S was in the off-site surgery center right before my surgery. He noted I had elected lumpectomy "*after* genetic testing, so you *knew* what you were choosing" with an edge in his voice. I do not know why. Here's something, though: Dr. S was in his element. I had never seen someone so at home in a health care setting. He whistled! He perfectly rendered the tune to "Hello! Ma Baby"—"Hello my baby, hello my honey, hello my ragtime gal." You may know the song and you may not. I know it from the Looney Tunes cartoon about the singing frog that tricks each man unlucky enough to find it. In the cartoon, a hapless everyman by chance finds a small box stuck inside a column or a wall. He opens the box and a frog jumps out, but not just any frog—this is a frog that can sing and dance, twirl a top hat, and artfully swing a cane, all while belting out, "Hello my baby, hello my honey, hello my ragtime gal," to the tune that Dr. S whistled away before my surgery.

It is a strange cartoon, dark really, a morality tale about greed and gullibility, because the frog was a tease. When the man sees the frog singing and dancing, his eyes light up with dollar signs: this frog will make his fortune! He rents an auditorium and sells enough tickets to fill it with listeners, opens the box holding the frog, and the frog jumps out but then does . . . nothing. It sits on the stage. Sometimes it ribbits. The audience becomes enraged and the man who found the frog grabs the frog and runs away, feeling lucky to escape with his life. While running he shoves the frog back in the box and stuffs the box into a new hiding place. Time passes until another luckless victim finds the frog, only to be duped in exactly the same way. Like the man in the cartoon, I found myself wondering whether Dr. S. was the real deal, or whether I had been duped by reports of his talent. I wanted to say: *Why are you whistling that dancing frog song before my surgery?* But really, I couldn't complain. I knew what I was getting, at least somewhat. I chose Dr. S over another surgeon recommended by my internist, a surgeon I had interviewed and found to be understanding and compassionate.

My friend U, who'd been diagnosed several months before I was, opted for that surgeon because his personal warmth and friendliness made her feel safe. I'll call that surgeon Dr. R. I met him. I liked him, but, unlike my friend, I did not find his soft edges reassuring, because I couldn't sense a hard-edged intelligence accompanying them. For my surgeon, I wanted a mind as sharp as the knives he used and when I met Dr. S, despite the oddness, that is what I thought I had found. Since my operation, many people have told me that Dr. S is "the best," and my scars are clean and healed well. He also got all the cancer the first time—my margins were, as they say, clean. Still, something in me was upset that day as I waited outside the operating room. Frustrated at his whistling, his inability to speak plainly, even the suggestion, or joke, in his office that my husband might be the bus driver. When I related all this to an MD friend, he asked me afterwards, "Theresa, why do you go to a surgeon?" "Um, for surgery?" I answered. Yes. That's right. For surgery.

Right before I left the surgical center, still half-asleep from the anesthetic, one of the nurses told me, or whispered in my ear—I remember only a voice—"Dr. S says women shouldn't need pain medicine. As if his technique is so good the patient won't feel pain." The voice paused, then resumed seconds later, even quieter this time, "But then again, Dr. S has never had his breast cut open."

Dr. S did his best work, some would say his most important work, when patients were asleep, and he did it very well. He also knew his stuff as far as the relevant surgical questions went: the value of genetic testing, reasons for a double mastectomy and that it should be my decision, not his. He practiced "shared decision-making," meaning the clinician presents options and gives patients guidance, but if there is a choice to be made that is truly a choice—about quality of life, more or less invasive procedures, more or less aggressive treatment—the patient decides. Dr. S did this. He did it in his own indirect, you-could-be-the-bus-driver way, but he did it, and I knew, from what his staff nurse told me, he was committed to it, not because he believed in "shared decision-making" as the flavor-of-the-month in surgical practice, but because it was the right way to approach difficult medical decisions. Moreover, I never felt rushed by him during that initial consultation. He wanted me to understand what my choices were and that they depended on the results of my genetic testing. Looked at objectively, Dr. S's discussion with me represented the gold standard of care. Indeed, I felt satisfied with him, very satisfied, when I left his office.

But after the surgery was done, I wanted him to be kinder. He had successfully steered me to genetic testing, finished the operation with clean margins, and confirmed (via pathology) that my lymph nodes were free of disease. Once all that was done, I wanted a surgeon who was more normal, less quirky. I wanted the friendly, reassuring surgeon, who would hold my hand and make me feel like a human being.

FOURTEEN

Not on the List

THE MORNING OF my surgery, Arthur and I drove to the surgical center where Dr. S worked on Fridays. It was located in a Pittsburgh suburb and I had reservations about having my surgery at a stand-alone center so far away from a hospital. If anything went wrong, where would the rapid response team come from, since there wasn't an ICU? I've seen too many actual in-hospital emergencies. However, we walked in and the calmness of the place soothed me. There were no clusters of tense people in the waiting room, no one rushing around, no repeated dings of elevators or intrusive overhead pages.

At the check-in desk, I gave my name, and the person standing behind the desk—I couldn't say if she was a tech, aide, nurse, or administrator—flipped through the multipage record of names and surgical-appointment times she held in her hand and, barely looking up, said, "You're not on the list." Just like that, she said it.

In our family, we joke about "the Nurse Voice." As in, "Don't make me use the Nurse Voice," the tone that insists, *You will do what I say.* The Nurse Voice is usually deployed on behalf of someone else, but that day I used it for myself. "I'd better be on the list." That was it, a statement of fact, but also a statement of, "If I'm not on the list *now*, I soon will be." And a statement of, "I'm having surgery *today.*"

She—whoever she was—picked up the list again and went through it, slightly more slowly than she had the first time, sliding her finger down the row of names before she flipped each page over. In the middle of her scrolling, she stopped: "You're on the list." She did not say, "Don't see how I missed you" or "Of course you're on the list" or "Sorry about that." My not being on the list seemed implausible. Do people come to surgical centers at eight in the morning on the wrong day? It's hard to believe that actually happens, especially since I didn't know my arrival time until the day before my operation, when someone from the surgical center called to confirm the date and tell me the time of my surgery.

Could it be that the computer system at the center often left patients off the list? That also seems unlikely, though the list looked hard to read. It was crammed with information and picking out individual names wasn't easy. Afterwards, I thought that patient names should be put in boldface to avoid mistakes by list-readers who rushed even when there was no reason to hurry. Someone could also have made a cover sheet with patients' names listed in alphabetical order and they could index that list to the longer, actual list that gave the times of surgeries. But then, right then, I suggested none of that. I stood at the check-in desk and looked at the woman holding the list. I stared at her.

It made no difference. She didn't care. I confess there is a part of me that wants to find that person again, back her up against a wall, get right in her face, and bellow in the Nurse Voice, "WHAT DO YOU MEAN I'M NOT ON THE LIST?" I am not given to violence, to wanting to hurt others. I have had patients yell at me, call me incompetent, and threaten me, and I never wanted to hurt them back. Never. But each time an incident like this happened during my cancer treatment, as with the "You just missed her" receptionist in mammography, I felt feral, in thought if not in deed. And it kept happening. I had not understood that indifference can become a form of cruelty when one's life could be at stake.

Thoughtless care is also bad practice. *Compassionomics: The Revolutionary Scientific Evidence that Caring Makes a Difference* argues that compassion has clinical benefits beyond simply making patients feel better about themselves and the care they receive. The authors, physicians Stephen Trzeciak and Anthony Mazzarelli, discuss multiple studies that show the positive physical effects of compassion. One study, done in the 1960s at Massachusetts General Hospital in Boston, found that preoperative patients who received an extra visit from the anesthesiologist prior to surgery needed less sedation before surgery and were significantly calmer than patients who did not have the extra visit. A similar study done in 2015 found that pre-op visits from surgical nurses trained in compassionate care led to patients ranking their postoperative pain 50 percent lower than patients who did not receive an extra nursing visit. The authors conclude: "In these randomized trials of vulnerable patients about to undergo surgery, the health care providers *themselves* made a major difference in the patients' care." Compassion also reduced the cost of care, since patients in the "compassion groups" needed less sedation and less pain medicine overall.

If compassion has measurable beneficial results, what must be the effect of compassionless care? Is there a significant negative effect from showing up for surgery and having the first person the patient sees blithely announce that she is "not on the list"? Since I wanted to back that person into a wall and yell right into her face—something I have never done, nor ever really wanted to do before that day—I would say yes. My blood pressure probably rose along with my levels of cortisol, a stress hormone. My heart rate likely increased along with my respirations and I felt a sense of panic: fight or flight—the sympathetic nervous system taking over. Maybe that's even what turned me against Dr. S's whistling and his mild aggression, what made me feel tense and besieged while I waited for surgery. My whole experience might have been different, better, if the person with the list had made an effort to be kind.

A few days after the surgery I received a Patient Satisfaction Survey via email. I tend to not like those surveys because in my view they focus attention on surface details. I would rather they collected patient impressions to really improve care by, say, getting the hospital to hire more nurses, or by strengthening communication between members of the health care team.

This time when I filled out the survey, though, I had something to say. I described being told I was not on the list of patients scheduled for surgery the day I came in. No one, I wrote, wants to hear that they are not on the list.

FIFTEEN

Theresa in Cancerland, Part I

THE OPENING LINES of Lewis Carroll's nonsense poem "Jabberwocky" sound like language after cancer. First, you cry. Then you get the diagnosis confirmed with a biopsy (or two) and a pathologist's report. Next you tell people. Then it's time for treatment. But before treatment can begin, the slowest two weeks in the history of time's passing go by while you wait for the results of genetic testing. Ordinary words cannot capture the feeling of being upside-down, stuck on the teeter-totter, seeing and sawing, but getting nowhere.

Here are the first four lines of "Jabberwocky":

> 'Twas brillig, and the slithy toves
> Did gyre and gimble in the wabe
> All mimsy were the borogoves,
> And the mome raths outgrabe.

This is nonsense. I think I get the meaning or at least I get an impression: it was sunny out, at the seaside, and animals called toves, borogroves, and raths play in the waves (wabe). My interpretation could be completely wrong, though, since the entire short poem is about a young boy on a quest to kill the monster known as the Jabberwock and the first four lines are the final four lines of the poem, too.

Cancer has not so much its own language, outside of health care, as its own meaning. I spoke the word "cancer" often as a nurse, discussed diagnoses with patients and talked over side effects of chemotherapy. But hearing the word "cancer" as a patient, as in "my cancer," I hear not English, but Lewis Carroll: "Beware the Jubjub bird, and shun / The frumious Bandersnatch!" Cancer as "frumious Bandersnatch!"—it makes sense, at least as much as anything else. The words, the nonsense, capture the meaning-shifting that happened when I was diagnosed with cancer. For example, genetic mutations are all represented by acronyms that look like codes. In addition to BRCA1 and 2, there's MLH1, MSH2 and 6, PMS2, PTEN, and APC for breast cancer, colon cancer, and familial adenomatosis polyposis. I read about these mutations when I learned how to calculate risk, but they have now become a sea of nonsensical capital letters in my head: *'Twas brillig, and the slithy toves.*

Even though I forgot practically everything I had ever learned about cancer when I became a cancer patient, I did remember one cold hard fact: patients died. I knew very little about mastectomy, and double mastectomy even less. I knew it as a mouthful, I knew that done prophylactically it was part of "the full Angelina Jolie." But I didn't know the details of it, literally in the flesh. I found those details online, though. There are pictures all over the internet of women who have had mastectomies and they show every stage along the way: women with puckered red skin where their breasts used to be, women stretching the skin of their breasts with expanders after mastectomy to accommodate breast implants, women who had nipple-preserving surgery, women who had roses tattooed over their mastectomy scars, women with nipples tattooed on to reconstructed breasts. One evening before our regular Sunday family dinner I was looking at those photos, making sad shocked noises. My daughter Miranda walked over and shut my laptop. "No, Mom," she said. "No more."

There was one photo I liked. A young woman, with short, straight blonde hair and a sly smile, wore a sleeveless white T-shirt that said, "Of course these are fake. My real ones tried to kill me." This looking—cancer voyeurism, perhaps—was what I did while I waited for the genetic testing results, since a mastectomy might be advisable depending on which mutations I had. Or rather, that's what I did when I couldn't help myself: surfed the internet for pictures of mastectomies. The medical websites that described mastectomy, even the ones I trusted, made surgery and reconstruction sound very straightforward. I wondered if the operations were straightforward for the surgeons, but afterwards not always for patients. Some sites described breast reconstruction after mastectomy as analogous to a woman being fully restored to her precancer self, or at least her precancer bust. A "famous hospital" website declared: "No longer do women need to face long, jagged scars that impact their self-image. Instead, advanced techniques have given plastic surgeons the tools to rebuild a woman's breast in such a way that her silhouette is once again whole." That sounds like a 1950s ad for a Maidenform bra. I have never thought of myself having a "silhouette" and never contemplated its "wholeness" being compromised in some dreadful way. I value my life a thousand times more than my silhouette and yet my bust seems to be what cancer threatens: "Beware the Jabberwock, my son! / The jaws that bite, the claws that catch!"

I own a small metal pillbox with a picture of a nurse on it. She's wearing an old-style white nurse's dress and of course a nurse's cap, and she says, with a friendly smile, "We prefer the term 'discomfort.'" I bought the pillbox because it made me laugh, and to remind myself that people in health care often minimize patients' distress. So, I didn't believe those calm clinical descriptions of mastectomy and reconstruction and I didn't even fully believe the women I talked to who had mastectomy and reconstruction and said the surgeries were fine, though I didn't tell them that. In *The Undying: Pain, Vulnerability, Mortality, Medicine, Art, Time, Dreams, Data, Exhaustion, Cancer, and Care*, poet and breast cancer patient Anne Boyer describes being sent home after having her mastectomy at an off-site surgical center. She wasn't even given an overnight in the hospital, and they discharged her with multiple drains hanging, pendulous, from her body.

Then there's breast cancer pink. I got my initial diagnosis at the end of August, and in October, the cotton-candy pink that has come to symbolize breast cancer was suddenly everywhere I went. A pink banner decorated an entire wall of the room where I had a diagnostic MRI. One of the buildings in downtown Pittsburgh illuminates its decorative top floors with pink lights for the entire month of October. In the past, the water in Pittsburgh's large downtown fountain has been dyed pink for October, a monthlong spewing that reminds me of the blood and tissue waste left behind after mastectomies. During a plane trip I took in the middle of the month, the flight attendants wore scarves decorated with swirls of pink. They also offered a pink drink: club soda and pink grapefruit juice, I think. Can you imagine? We clink a toast to breast cancer pink.

Susan G. Komen for the Cure is responsible for the ubiquity of the breast-cancer-as-pink symbology. Opinions about the Komen organization are mixed. Some people think Komen has done a lot of good by promoting screening mammography. Others argue that much of their money could have been better spent on research into the causes of and treatments for breast cancer. Some cancer bloggers fault Komen for not fully addressing the lack of a cure for metastatic breast cancer and for ignoring patients who are dying of breast cancer. But for me, it's the pink. The pink is irksome. Nancy Brinker, who founded Komen after the 1980 breast cancer death of her thirty-six-year-old sister, Susan Komen, argued in a letter to the *New York Times* that pink was her sister's favorite color and the Komen organization would continue to use the color pink to represent breast cancer for that reason. She wrote this letter in response to my *New York Times* column "Breast Cancer Is Serious, Pink Is Not."

To me, pink equals femininity, and being diagnosed with breast cancer made me fear for my life, not my sense of whether I would still be feminine enough—whatever that means—following my treatment. It's worth quoting a section of the column here to make the point that women diagnosed with breast cancer worry about dying:

> Being preoccupied with saving one's life produces a myopia, in which other worries unrelated to one's possibly imminent death fall away . . . I did ask my husband, "If I lose my breasts, will you love me the same way?" I was half-joking, but the question was also ridiculous because I knew the answer. Knew it: "Yes." Still, I feel that my asking it resulted from a kind of primordial sexism that, despite my best efforts, continues to infect my thoughts. The association of femininity and breast cancer is pernicious, because it genders the disease, meaning that a diagnosis of breast cancer marks patients as women first, people second. It implies that our womanliness is diseased, not our bodies.

I have never met an actual breast cancer patient who likes the pink. Never. They may be out there—but I don't know them. So I'm asking. Could we have a new color? Or no color at all? Why does breast cancer need a color to pretty it up, like a pink ribbon tied around a pony's tail or woven through a little girl's braids? It is not necessary, when one receives a breast cancer diagnosis, to emphasize a symbol that announces, *Hey, in case you missed it, I'm a woman.* Or, in our most current language, to suggest that breast cancer compromises my ability to successfully identify as female, and to avoid that threat I must decorate myself with pink. The color of cancer, any cancer, more likely resembles the fire that the Jabberwock sees with: "The Jabberwock, with eyes of flame . . . burbled as it came!" "Burbled" like a threatening monster, or a pink fountain, or club soda being poured into a glass half-filled with ice and pink grapefruit juice. If breast cancer has to have a color, for god's sake, it absolutely should not be pink.

There's also something called postmastectomy pain syndrome (PMPS): "The jaws that bite, the claws that catch!" Dr. S never mentioned PMPS to me, which might seem unsurprising since I did not have a mastectomy, but you can get it with lumpectomy, too. I know about PMPS because I am pretty sure I have it. I will, occasionally—every few weeks or so—have a random burst of very sharp pain at my surgical scar. It feels like someone inside my chest has a knife they are trying poke out of my body, through my incision site. It's thought that PMPS is caused by the regrowth of nerve cells, so maybe the pain is a good sign. I'm not sure. Oh, and for several months after my lumpectomy, my armpit was numb. Apparently, that's normal, too, but no one told me that either. Having that pain is, no question, better than being dead from cancer. Ditto for the numb armpit. But "pain" and "survival" do not sit on opposite ends of the seesaw, with survival holding pain off the ground, weightless and irrelevant.

Remember the patient who had her port removed on the Fourth of July? The alternative to a port is a different kind of surgically implanted central line that typically leaves the patient with three separate tubes hanging from his chest. Unlike the port, this type of central line can be used to give patients three different intravenous infusions at once, making it easy to manage complex oncological care. But that kind of implanted intravenous line, also unlike the port, gives bacteria three very accessible doors to the body, so the surgical site where the device exits the chest has to be covered at all times with an airtight dressing that gets replaced every week (what my young, impatient patient needed). To shower, the patient has to cover the dressing to keep the external tubes from getting wet, and when I worked at the hospital, leukemia and lymphoma patients were discharged from the hospital to return home with their central lines in place. They would need additional scheduled doses of chemo, plus fluids, and a central line is the safest way to do both at once.

These implanted, multipronged intravenous catheters made the care we gave more fluid—pun not intended. But not once did I think about what an annoyance a central line must be, especially once a patient is discharged to home. In my blinkered view, hospital patients were patients *only*. They needed central lines for as long as possible so that we could treat them as effectively as possible, even outside the hospital, and therefore they went home with their central lines. But my patients, I now realize after having been one myself, wanted to see themselves as regular people. "Patient" did not denote who they were. The central line with its plastic tubes protruding from their chests must have been a constant reminder of their disease, similar to my having PMPS. It forced them, and me, to remember that survival came with trade-offs.

But we saved their life. We nurses said it to one another all the time, to brush off a complaint—about her hair falling out, or that he'd lost his sense of taste, or how hard it was to take a shower with parts of a central line that shouldn't get wet hanging out of one's upper chest. At the time it wasn't meant as a brush-off either, but as a way of highlighting value: *We saved patients' lives.* The mistake we made was in thinking that the good made the bad unimportant, trivial, beside the point. It doesn't. *'Twas brillig, and the slithy toves*: Patients might as well have been saying that to me for all I grasped of their ordinary pain. At the end of every shift, I went home with my hair on my head and the skin of my chest intact. I took a normal shower, never giving a second thought to how easy it was.

As a patient, though, I contemplated the removal of both my breasts because a mistake in my genetic code would make a double mastectomy prudent. During the period of waiting for the genetic testing results, someone whom I won't identify said to Arthur, "I'm sure everything will be fine," when talking about me. How could they know? No one knew, including Dr. S. It was the weekend and Arthur and I went for a bike ride, but I kept hearing *I'm sure everything will be fine* repeat in my head until it became so overwhelming that I had to stop pedaling. Suddenly, I wanted to throw my bike down the hill bordering the path, wanted to mangle it to match the mangling of my fears, for *mangle* means "mutilate," but also "to create incoherence," as in the mangling of a text or a concern.

This anger I felt—anger that I didn't act on but that made me want to hurt people, break things—arose from helplessness. I was an angry child, or so said my parents, sometimes about moments in my childhood that I was too young to remember. Being a mom myself, I know that children's rage usually has a cause. For me, it came down to feeling less important than my older brother, who was born just sixteen months before I was. I don't think anyone consciously regarded me as lesser, and I'm not sure what my brother would say about this, but I felt I was of lowlier status—a very personal sense of injustice.

Also, my parents divorced when I was ten and my dad's involvement with the woman who became my stepmother, the woman who later lit her hair on fire, was revealed. Ten-year-old me believed that she, or he and she together, broke up the marriage, broke my home. It's hard to imagine how a child could not be angry about that. Now that I'm older and married, I see how different my parents are from each other and find it hard to imagine them ever being married to each other, but losing one's family unit is an injury.

During my childhood I was often told, "You can control your anger." Was this because my anger was inconvenient, or because I was a girl? Rage, ire, fury, indignation, wrath—girls and women are not supposed to show these emotions. That's why English has the words *bitch*, *shrew*, *scold*, *fishwife*, *fury*, *gorgon*, *harridan*, *harpy*, *termagant*, and *virago*. Monikers reserved for women.

The most helpful essay I have read on women's anger was written by Leslie Jamison, author of *The Empathy Exams*, and is titled "I Used to Insist I Didn't Get Angry. Not Anymore. On Female Rage." I wonder if it took a woman who had written an entire book on empathy to explicate "female rage," and to clarify that only by first exhibiting compassion for ourselves can women accept that we, too, can be mad as hell. This is what Jamison calls "an owning of accountability." The essay probes the writings of Aristotle, Martha Nussbaum, and Audre Lorde, in addition to discussing the presentation of anger by celebrities such as Uma Thurman and Tonya Harding. In the end Jamison concludes that her own newly recognized anger is not sufficient unto itself—it demands a response: "A vision of anger as fuel and fire, as a powerful inoculation against passivity . . . This anger is more like an itch than a wound. It demands that something *happen*."

Yes; that I understand. And what did I want to happen? As a child I wanted to feel like an equal member of the family. As a cancer patient I wanted the people taking care of me to be kinder and I wanted friends and family—most, but not all of whom were wonderful—to grasp that cancer sounds to the patient like a death sentence, or at least it did to me. There is no "everything will be fine" until everything actually is once again fine, if it ever is. Being angry made me feel that I could, if only briefly, triumph over people's insensitivity, the ubiquitous pink, all those proliferating acronyms.

However, the sense of victory never lasted long, because cancer, like the Jabberwock, is a monster and a maker of nonsense. Surgery kills the monster by cutting it out: "The vorpal blade went snicker-snack!" But in the meantime, the reality of having the disease can make the world absurd.

'Twas brillig, and the slithy toves / Did gyre and gimble in the wabe. "We prefer the term 'discomfort.'" "Her silhouette is once again whole." THINK PINK! "I'm sure everything will be fine." *Treatment saved your life.* "Of course these are fake. My real ones tried to kill me."

SIXTEEN

Theresa in Cancerland, Part II

AFTER MY BREAST cancer diagnosis, I never saw the rabbit holes coming. I knew that Google had answers, of course, but Google is more than a rabbit hole. Google leads straight to the Jabberwock—the nonsense monster. I have known cancer patients, and their loved ones, who caused themselves immense pain by turning to Google for answers to their cancer questions. There are some safe sites: the American Cancer Society, the National Cancer Institute, the CDC. There are also multiple breast cancer blogs and chat rooms that are not attached to organizations, as well as websites sponsored by pharmaceutical companies, which the companies use to advertise their cancer drugs. To be trustworthy, a cancer website needs to be disinterested, as in impartial, not seeking personal advantage. A blog, a chat room, even a site sponsored by a drug company, may have useful information, but I felt I could trust few that I looked at.

So, one of the first decisions I made following my cancer diagnosis was to adhere to an online blackout except for what

I considered purely scientific questions. My adherence wasn't 100 percent, as evidenced by my looking up mastectomy pictures online, but as much as I could, I avoided surfing the web. Instead of opening myself up to the overproliferation of possibly biased information on Google—the flood of nonsense I wanted to avoid—I searched for research articles that addressed specific concerns I had. I would learn about my disease from peer-reviewed articles in medical journals that discussed data. That felt safe.

Data about what, though? About which types of breast cancer? There are several kinds. The majority are similar to mine: positive for the hormones estrogen and progesterone (ER+/PR+) and negative for human epidermal growth factor receptor 2 (called HER2-, or Herceptin, after the drug used to treat it). This kind of breast cancer responds well to treatment and some women don't need chemotherapy. If there is such a thing as catching a break with cancer, then I caught that break. Another type of breast cancer is somewhat less easily treated: ER+/PR+ and HER2+. That type tends to be more aggressive and treatment usually includes using Herceptin. Herceptin is a monoclonal antibody, an artificially created molecule that binds to HER2 receptors on the tumor, stopping its out-of-control growth. There are also triple-negative breast cancers (TNBC), which lack receptors for estrogen, progesterone, and human epidermal growth factor receptor 2 (ER-/PR-/HER2-). Approximately 10 to 15 percent of women are diagnosed with TNBC every year and historically this type of breast cancer is very difficult to treat and has a worse prognosis than the "positive" kinds. Anne Boyer, the poet who wrote the Pulitzer

Prize–winning book *The Undying*, had triple-negative breast cancer.

Are you confused yet? The location of the tumor also matters for diagnosis. DCIS stands for ductal carcinoma in situ, meaning the cancer stayed localized in a mammary gland or duct. Breast cancers that are not "in situ" are called "invasive," a terrifying word when used to describe a cancer. It means that the cancer spread to breast tissue outside a mammary gland. My cancer was invasive and DCIS, denoting that it had broken out of the milk duct by the time it was discovered on the ultrasound. The two different labels—*DCIS* and *invasive*—confused me when I first read the pathologist's report. I thought I had two different cancers, but it was the same cancer that had burst its original bounds.

Complicating matters, some advocates against overtreatment of breast cancer insist that DCIS is not really cancer, but should instead be considered a sort of maybe-cancer that might never cause harm. My friend H, the oncology nurse practitioner, said they call DCIS "zero stage" cancer, but when I brought up the dismissiveness with which I've heard DCIS described vis-à-vis the health threat it poses, she responded, "Well, we definitely take it seriously." The two women I know who had DCIS very much feel that they had cancer.

Getting into the anatomy of it, breasts have lobules, where milk is made, as well as ducts to transport the milk, and lobular breast cancer is another separate type of breast cancer. Similar to ductal breast cancer, lobular breast cancer also comes in contained and invasive forms, called respectively lobular carcinoma in situ (LCIS) and invasive lobular carcinoma (ILC).

According to the Lobular Breast Cancer Alliance, ILC is "the sixth most frequently diagnosed cancer of women in the US," and yet even though I worked in oncology as a nurse and have had a lifetime fear of and fascination with breast cancer, I never would have heard of lobular carcinoma if not for hearing about a friend of a friend who was diagnosed with ILC, and had it successfully treated.

There's also inflammatory breast cancer, a rare and aggressive form of the disease that presents differently from most other breast cancers. Inflammatory breast cancer typically has a high mortality rate and a short life expectancy compared to other breast cancers. However, as of this writing, nurse and palliative care activist Amy Berman, a senior program officer with the John A. Hartford Foundation in New York City, is still alive and working full-time following her diagnosis of inflammatory breast cancer in 2010. I know Amy's story well because I wrote about her in the *New York Times*, in a piece entitled "When the Patient Knows Best."

Each kind of breast cancer comes with its own risk of recurrence, based on whether or not the disease returned in women who all had the same disease, and it's rare, but men get breast cancer, too. According to the National Cancer Institute (NCI): "Male breast cancer makes up less than 1 percent of all cases of breast cancer." The NCI says that there were an estimated 268,600 new cases of breast cancer in women in 2019, which means that around 2,600 men also got breast cancer that year. And while no men have been diagnosed with lobular carcinoma in situ, men can get DCIS, invasive ductal carcinoma, inflammatory breast cancer, and a rare form of breast cancer that also affects women, called Paget's disease of the nipple. The men who get breast cancer tend to be in their sixties and seventies, and I can only imagine how hard it might be for them to disclose their diagnosis.

This reminds me of another rare cancer: adenoid cystic carcinoma (ACC). This type of cancer is usually found in salivary glands, but sometimes it grows in the breast (and other locations as well). When a pathologist examines ACC cells that were biopsied from a woman's breast, those cells will not look like breast cancer. They will appear instead like adenoid cystic carcinoma cells. The cancer did not travel to the breast from the salivary glands, but for some reason as yet unknown, this glandular cancer sometimes starts up in the breast, rather than its normal biological location.

Are you even more confused?

A real rabbit hole is a home, a warren, but I did not feel at home going down these cancer information tunnels. It should have been easy for me to find statistics on my risk of recurrence, data that would say how likely it was for my particular cancer to return. The risk was very low, I knew, and maybe that should have been enough, but I wanted to see the statistics for myself, read the papers on my own. Yet I could not find any one article that exclusively referred to my situation, in part due to the way that patient data was aggregated in research studies. One study that followed breast cancer patients whose tumors had my specific tumor markers (ER+/PR+, HER2-) didn't divide patients into whether they were pre- or postmenopausal at diagnosis, even though that's a relevant distinction. In general, breast cancers diagnosed before menopause tend to be more aggressive than those diagnosed after. Mine was diagnosed right before, and I tell myself that my own proximity to menopause takes the edge off some of that premenopausal breast cancer aggressiveness, even though, as far as I know, nothing in physiology or breast cancer research gives credence to the protective effect of "near menopause"—a term I myself made up after being diagnosed.

While I'm talking about menopause, I'll take a moment to mention the self-disclosure rabbit hole. I never thought I would write a book about my breasts (or specifically my right breast). The subject of *breast* cancer feels more revealing, in a way, than talking about my fear of death, my unexpected rage, and my new-found awareness of how often I failed, as a nurse, to fully appreciate how burdened my patients were by their illnesses. Breasts are personal, private, but the Centers for Disease Control reports that breast cancer is the second leading cause of cancer deaths among most American women, and the most common cause of cancer deaths for women of Hispanic origin. I disclose medical details about my life to show what I learned from having cancer, but it makes me feel exposed, as if my story comes in a string bikini top. It feels as if I'm showing off my breasts, or breast, inappropriately to everyone, a behavior choice I would generally view negatively.

Back to the research rabbit hole. I'm worried that my cancer will defy the odds, come back with a vengeance, and kill me. That's why I wanted data just for me—not with pre- and postmenopausal women combined, not with women who are BRCA1 and BRCA2 positive mixed up with those who aren't, not with triple-negative women tossed into the mix, not with women who were stage II or stage III grouped together with my stage I. I don't want those women, with their statistically higher rates of recurrence, rubbing shoulders with me. I don't want anyone's genetic proclivity to an aggressive cancer to make my chances look worse than they are.

Stop a minute. You know I'm fooling myself here, right? What I really wanted was to find a statistical home for my cancer anxiety, a warren where I could store my fear. Instead, one hole led to another, paths connected up at unexpected points, and ended when I wanted them to go on, or kept going when I had already learned more than I could handle. That home doesn't exist. I might search every six months or even every six days for that elusive data-just-for-me, but in the end, it wouldn't help. No expertly aggregated, perfectly calibrated, soothingly informative, and confidently reassuring data was out there.

I suggest patients not go down the cancer rabbit hole. There's nothing wholly good there and I wish I had expanded my internet ban to include research articles and, well, pretty much anything about cancer, including the mastectomy photos I couldn't keep myself from looking at. A warren is a home, but it can also be a labyrinth or maze. I went looking for hope in the internet's twists and turns, its dark passages and unexpected dead ends. But I only found more sustenance for my fears, which already bred like rabbits.

SEVENTEEN

Nature/Nurture

I WOULD LIKE to say that I do not cry easily. It's a point of pride among many nurses. Work is not for crying, and if a nurse cries while on duty at the hospital, the situation must be bad. I cried the day of my diagnostic ultrasound, when the radiologist told me, "I see a mass," but after that I only occasionally shed tears over having cancer.

Two of those times I remember very well because they happened in the same place: Pittsburgh's Frick Park. At 644 acres, Frick is the largest park in Pittsburgh and makes you feel as if you're in a forest even though you're in the middle of the city. The first crying incident happened shortly after the follow-up ultrasound, before my diagnosis was confirmed, when part of me hoped that the radiologist had been wrong, even though most of me believed she was right. Arthur and I went for a walk in the park. It was a nice autumn weekend and the winding paths were unusually crowded with people wanting to enjoy the sunny fall day.

Rates of cancer survival are often tabulated in five-year increments and while walking I suddenly felt what it would be like if my life ended in five years. Miranda and Sophia would have just finished college. Conrad would be finishing his PhD in economics. Probably none of them would be married and there would be no grandchildren (if they chose to marry and have children). I stopped and stood as tears rolled down my face. How, in five years, could I no longer be part of their lives, hear about their successes and concerns, buck them up if they were troubled, comfort them in sadness? It was as if a great gulf appeared, and the part of my future that would have been filled with the children as they aged and changed, held nothing. It was the saddest feeling I have ever known.

Arthur stopped, looked at my face, and pulled me off the path since it was full of walkers. I felt that same self-consciousness I had felt at the hospital, crying in the hallway with other women getting mammograms. What would people think I was crying about? And then I didn't care what they thought. *Five years. Five years.* My life over in five years.

The feeling passed as I took shelter in rationality: don't worry before there's a definitive diagnosis. But that fear left a mark. My mortality isn't mine alone—my death would affect the people in the world I love the most, including Arthur, too, of course.

THE OTHER TIME I cried in Frick Park happened when I was almost done with radiation. Arthur and I were walking, on a different path, this time with our dog. It was a bright mid-December day, cool, but not cold. The trees were bare of leaves, but the grass remained green and the sunlight in late afternoon was so bright I had to turn my eyes away. I wanted to explain to Arthur how I felt, that suddenly I feared dying, but I couldn't make my feelings clear. I decided to keep walking on my own, wanting only myself for company. Arthur and the dog kept going on a separate path, and I sat down on a park bench and cried deep, heaving sobs. No one else was there, but part of me wished someone were, to put their arms around me, as the ultrasound tech had done, and say, *You will survive this.*

No one came. Time passed and I stopped crying, but still felt cancer's shadow. The park's greenery, the sun, made no difference. I started walking though, and the familiar dirt paths and blinding but enlivening sunlight had their effect. I hiked upwards, following a new route from the one we started out on, going back to the beginning, and soon I felt calmer. It came to seem unlikely that I would die that day, or even the day after.

As she was dying of cancer, poet Audre Lorde wrote in *The Marvelous Arithmetics of Distance*:

Today is not the day.

It could be

But it is not.

Today is today.

I read that poem before I ever had cancer, quoted those lines of poetry in a monthly newsletter I wrote for cancer patients when I worked at the hospital. *Today is today.* Could brilliance be more obvious or more simple? Cancer is cancer, but today is today.

I walked home. I don't remember the walk—it was so familiar after all, and I was deep in thought. My today, plus the day after.

EIGHTEEN

Chemo: Yes or No

IT USED TO be that every woman with my kind of breast cancer got chemotherapy. Well, actually, it used to be that every woman got a mastectomy. Then research proved that lumpectomy offered similarly good results in terms of recurrence risk if it was paired with other treatments, typically chemotherapy and radiation—the cancer trifecta of cut, poison, burn.

There is probably no health care treatment more dreaded than chemotherapy, thanks in part to the way its side effects are portrayed in plays, movies, and television shows about cancer patients. Patients lose their hair. There's vomiting, lots of vomiting. The infusion centers depicted on TV are invariably impersonal and depressing. Cancer treatment comes across as a physical and emotional endurance test and chemo is the hardest part. The truth is both less immediately theatrical and worse than typically portrayed, because those side effects afflict real people.

I, however, might not need it. *I might not need it.* Data can now tell oncologists whether certain breast cancer patients will benefit from chemo. There's a test, called Oncotype DX, that reveals whether chemotherapy actually reduces a woman's risk of a cancer recurrence, and each test costs about $3,000. Before my surgery, someone, I can't remember who, told me that I wouldn't need chemotherapy. It must have been Dr. S, right? Who else would it have been? After the surgery, at a follow-up appointment with Dr. S's physician assistant, I was told "they"—whoever that meant—would determine whether chemo should be part of my treatment. Chemo was back on the table and the physician assistant was unprepared for how much that news would throw me. She also had no timeline for finding out if I needed chemo and she couldn't explain the process, beyond saying that the medical oncologist—the cancer doc who manages pharmaceutical treatment for cancer—and the surgeon would make the decision together. Radiation, which I knew I needed, came after chemo, if I had chemo. The treatment schedule in my head had included surgery, several weeks of postoperative recovery to give my skin time to heal, and then four weeks of daily radiation, after which active treatment would be over. My hope was to finish in time for Christmas. The PA's suggestion that I might need chemo alarmed me on its own and wrecked my schedule, shredding my plan to finish cancer treatment in a couple of months.

I didn't have a medical oncologist yet, or rather, following the schedule that had originally been discussed with me, I had an appointment with one, but it was six weeks away, when I thought radiation would be done. I now needed a medical oncologist immediately to tell me whether I needed chemo, and in Pittsburgh the medical oncologists were all booked up.

It was a classic catch-22. I couldn't get in to see a medical oncologist for several weeks, and I couldn't start radiation until the medical oncologist decided whether I needed chemotherapy. Back in what I call my past life as an English professor, I taught *Catch-22*, the satirical World War II novel by Joseph Heller, to freshmen at Tufts University. This brilliantly absurd book is set at a U.S. military base on an island in the Mediterranean Sea near Italy. Yossarian, the putative hero of the novel, and a bombardier, increasingly fears for his life as he accumulates ever larger numbers of successful bombing missions. His commanding officer, Colonel Cathcart, keeps upping the number of bombing missions each American soldier must complete before he is relieved from serving on future flights over Italy. As soon as a soldier gets close to the required number of missions, the colonel adds to that number, ensuring that soldiers continue risking their lives in dangerous bombing raids with no chance of a reprieve.

In the novel, commanding officers determine whether a bombing mission is needed by consulting a map of Italy posted in the soldiers' briefing room. On this map, a line indicates the enemy's location relative to the Allied Forces, and that line's position determines whether the Americans will go out on a mission. At one point, Yossarian sneaks into the briefing room in the middle of the night and *moves the line on the map*. The next morning, an official reading of the newly placed line leads to all bombing missions for the day being canceled. This episode confounded my students. "That wouldn't actually work, would it?" one asked. "You can't just move a line on a map and change what's real." Ah, but this is the point of satire. A real army would presumably rely on more than a single line on a map to authorize bombing raids during a war. But in *Catch-22*, Yossarian's desperate moving of the line accomplishes his goal because the military leaders in the novel are lazy and have no imagination. They can't conceive that Yossarian could use their own tricks against them.

I thought about the moving of the line and asked my students, "What if someone taped a note on the door to this room that said class was canceled. Would you believe it?" They would. This was before cell phones and group texts. A note on the door would efficiently communicate with the entire class and there would be no easy way to verify that it was real.

The research I did while waiting to see the oncologist suggested that determining whether chemo would benefit someone with my diagnosis could be quick. Despite my own warnings about the fear-stimulating effects of research, this was the one rabbit hole that proved useful. The Oncotype DX test requires a biopsy sample from the tumor and it takes about two weeks to get the results of the test. However, because the test is expensive, other oncologists have developed algorithms, formulaic clinical decision trees, that offer a close approximation of the test without using the test itself. One well-known algorithm was developed here in Pittsburgh and is called Magee Equations.

For the Magee Equations there are six required fields of information, including tumor size and positive or negative HER2 status. Anyone can enter the requested values into the appropriate fields and get a result. Interpreting the result can be complicated, although the decision-tree that accompanies the "equations" is easy to follow, at least for me, a nurse. The web page comes with a disclaimer that "The Magee Equations should only be used by medical professionals who understand its usefulness and limitations." I read this as the "don't sue us if your doctor disagrees with the result" clause.

I started to feel desperate about not knowing if I would need chemo and when I would be done with treatment. When I approached the medical oncologist I had an appointment with in six weeks, her office told me they absolutely would not let me come in earlier for the chemotherapy decision. This doctor was supposedly an expert in holistic care and I told her assistant that refusing to see me now, to resolve this one treatment question, felt completely nonholistic, but that didn't help me. So, I used my connections and asked an oncologist friend (not a breast cancer specialist) if he could help me get in to see a medical oncologist soon. I hated jumping the line, but Arthur wanted that and I had probably done it already, if not so overtly, with Dr. S.

I got in to see the doc I wanted early the next week, although not due to my oncologist friend's intervention, according to him. He said the office had already made an appointment for me following Arthur's phone call a few days before. At my first appointment I thanked the oncologist and her staff for getting me in so quickly. She demurred, and then turned the computer screen around so that I could see her enter my numbers into the Magee Equations. She coauthored one of the papers validating the equations but didn't bring that up. I didn't bring it up either, though I couldn't say why. The Magee Equations result was that, no, I would not need chemo, the answer I had suspected because I had already used the equations on my own computer. The process in the doctor's office, including turning the computer around and entering the numbers, took less than five minutes.

Here's how it felt, though: It felt like my oncologist moved the line. A line, an inflexible barrier had kept me from getting a timely and official answer to the question of whether I needed chemotherapy. One of the medical oncologists Arthur and I contacted had insisted through her assistant that making the chemo decision was very involved and took time. For my cancer and my oncologist—whom I'll call Dr. Y after Yossarian—that was not true. I know I was being the person no one in health care likes, the so-called "difficult patient" who won't take no for an answer and wants everything done NOW. For some breast cancer patients, though, the decision about needing chemo is not complicated if a validated algorithm or genetic test can be used to make the determination. Why should an answer that can be given in five minutes require a six-week wait?

Some might say that the high-tech nature of cancer treatment leads to such impersonal care. Philosopher Michel Foucault explored how science impacted the development of modern health care in *The Birth of the Clinic: An Archaeology of Medical Perception*. In describing the emergence of modern medicine in the eighteenth century, Foucault argued that as diseases were rigorously studied and objectively classified, the patient inevitably became less important than the disease itself: "Paradoxically, in relation to that which he is suffering from, the patient is only an external fact; the medical reading must take him into account only to place him in parentheses."

Foucault does not posit an unfeeling medical science against a vulnerable and devalued human body, though. He argues that many of the principles embraced in the French Revolution influenced the development of modern health care, so that as the practice of medicine became scientifically precise, it also strove to be respectful, empathic, and economically fair: "A certain balance must be kept, of course, between the interests of knowledge and those of the patient; there must be no infringement of the natural rights of the sick, or of the rights that society owes the poor."

The rights of the sick and the poor don't come up a lot in contemporary discussions about health care, at least in the U.S. We hear instead about the importance of relative value units (RVUs), diagnosis-related groups (DRGs), doing more with less, and maximizing profits. The present system values individuals in terms of the money they bring in—whether provider or patient. Nurses have a perverse kind of negative value because our salaries and benefits cost money but we don't generate income. This is why nurses are often overworked. Science and technology are not deforming health care, making it unwieldy and impersonal; greed is. The difficult patient attempts to yell her way through the noise of health care profiteering, saying, "Me, me, me! Help me, please!" Sometimes it works and other times it doesn't.

Once when I was a nurse in the hospital, a patient came in for scheduled chemo. Most people hate being in the hospital, and this patient acutely felt that way. His pretreatment clinical work—drawing labs, checking his weight, making sure his central line worked—had been done at the outpatient clinic across the street from the hospital before he even arrived on the floor. The idea was to start his chemotherapy quickly, as soon as he got put in a room if possible.

The nurses at the outpatient clinic were also supposed to start him on intravenous fluids, but he did not come to our hospital floor hooked up to a bag of IV saline, rolling a pump along on its wheeled pole. This meant that I needed to request an IV pump from supply, who would deliver it to the floor. Except when I called supply they told me they had no IV pumps— none—which was hard for me to believe, but I didn't go down to check, and why would they lie? No IV pump, no IV fluids, no chemo, no exceptions. Meanwhile, the patient stood in the doorway to his room, giving me hard looks whenever he caught my eye. Tall and thin, close to middle age, with short, spiky dark hair, he made his impatience obvious.

A couple of hours went by. The charge nurse asked me what the hold-up with the chemo was and I said I couldn't get an IV pump from supply—that they said there were no pumps. She answered sourly, "I've never heard that reason for not giving chemo," which may have been true, but it didn't help get me a pump. It was as if I were a bombardier ordered to go on a mission when no planes were available, and my failure to follow orders was being held against me. In other words, another catch-22. And that day, I didn't have it in me to scour the hospital looking for an available IV pump on a pole. I called supply repeatedly, and heard the same thing, every time: we don't have any pumps. So, I waited for an IV pump to be delivered to the floor. Usually in the hospital I would move heaven and earth for patients, or at least try, but this time, the patient's hallway glares, the outpatient clinic's failure to do their job, the bizarre shortage of a common piece of hospital equipment, all left me exhausted. My other patients were also keeping me busy.

When I became a cancer patient, I learned how it felt to be one among many. One more person caught in the giant health care revolving door. Except I wasn't one more person—I was me, frightened and alone receiving treatment that felt like DIY cancer care, as in do-it-yourself. Set up your own biopsy and hassle people to get the results. Find a surgeon. Find a medical oncologist. Find a radiation oncologist. Find the Magee Equations and fill them out. Find a new medical oncologist who is immediately available. Get so exasperated from making phone calls—phone calls!—that Arthur has to take over. I was a bone-marrow transplant nurse and a hospice nurse. I know how to get things done, but this, this DIY cancer care, was too much, even for me, an in-the-know expert in the field. Imagine if I didn't have the education and training that I have, the helpful husband, and yes, the strong sense that I, and everyone else, deserve better.

That day in the hospital when I could not get an IV pump, my patient may have felt aggrieved at his DIY cancer care. "What does someone have to do around here to get chemotherapy? Bring their own goddamn IV pump?" he might have asked rhetorically. He also might have been frightened and any security he felt about his course of treatment or controlling his disease or trusting his nurses and doctors probably took a big hit that day. All that, due to the inexplicable lack of a working IV pump in a hospital supply department usually filled with them. Oh, and a nurse who, one day out of many, felt unable to try harder to make a difficult patient's care happen.

NINETEEN

RadOnc

IT'S ONE WORD and the *a* is long: rād / onk. If you want to sound in-the-know, this is what you say for Radiation Oncology. It's also got a spondaic rhythm pattern (former English professor), which means both syllables are stressed. How's that for irony? Even the syllables are stressed in radiation oncology.

RadOnc doesn't stand alone. There's MedOnc, too, and SurgOnc. Orthopods for bones, ID for infectious disease. But there's something about RadOnc—what it signifies. Cut, poison, burn. I'd been cut before my lumpectomy, so I knew what that was like. I'd given patients chemo and seen it, mostly, help them. But I'd never been burned, or burned others. To me, RadOnc was an unknown.

My treatment began the Monday after Thanksgiving. I would go five days a week for four weeks and be done by Christmas; it was the schedule I had hoped for, with my treatments sandwiched between the two holidays. The radiologist came across as frank and caring. She stressed how important it was not to miss any days of treatment. Afterwards, a nurse talked to me about taking care of my skin. They wanted me to use aloe vera gel to keep my skin from burning, but I'm allergic to aloe so she said I could use Aquaphor instead and that I should apply it twice each day to the site on my breast—my right breast—that received the radiation. She apologized for not having any Aquaphor to offer me—most patients received a free bottle of aloe vera gel—but said I could get it at any drugstore.

I asked the doctor and the nurse about riding my bike to my treatments. Would that be a problem? They must have said no, because I rode my bike. The nurse might have said something about the Aquaphor becoming gloppy and extra messy if I got sweaty, but I think I made that up based on what riding my bike while using Aquaphor was like. Someone asked how far my house was from the hospital and the answer, "three miles," seemed acceptable.

Before I left RadOnc that day, they gave me an iPad to watch a video that showed what would happen during my treatments. Arthur was at the appointment with me, and we literally put our heads together to watch. As I recall, the video was straightforward, kind of boring even, but reassuring. It made radiation therapy seem almost ordinary, and the large machines looked like something out of a science fiction movie—not a scary movie like *Alien*, but a movie where everything more or less turns out OK in the end. It's interesting that I trusted this video and its presentation of radiation treatment's ordinariness, but mistrusted women's accounts of "ordinary" mastectomies and breast reconstruction. It makes sense when you think about it, though—videos of those actual surgical procedures would never come across as ordinary, but there are no laser beams or pictures of singed flesh to see with radiation therapy; most of the damage to cancer and the body is internal and therefore invisible.

After I met the doctor and the nurse and watched the video, I had another separate appointment where a technician took the measurements needed for my treatments. The technician looked and acted like no one else I have met working in health care. She was fairly short, and her long, fluffy hair and shaggy bangs formed a mane around her face. She cackled when she laughed and she made a series of ribald comments about revealing my breasts, having an audience see my breasts, etc. while she worked. Her jokes were crude and funny and I laughed the whole way through the session.

After taking my measurements she showed me the specially made shirts that RadOnc patients get for radiation therapy. "Volunteers make them," she said proudly as I looked at a rack of singularly hideously patterned short-sleeved shirts decorated with neon pentagrams inside dull pink squares and large avocado and cerise-colored flowers on backgrounds of dull brown. Imagine that Maria, the singing governess from *The Sound of Music*, found some really ugly drapes to use to sew shirts for cancer patients, instead of the lively flower prints from which she made clothing for the von Trapp children. No one would sing "Do-Re-Mi" in a field of Alpine flowers in one of those shirts.

I looked through them, each one uglier than the one before, and I loved them. First, they fastened with Velcro and the Velcro made the shirts special. Velcro connected the two front and side pieces of the shirt, making it easy to expose one breast for treatment and then put the shirt back together when treatment was done. I also liked how aggressively garish and dated the patterns on the shirts were, the opposite of the bland gowns patients usually wear. The third thing to like: the shirts opened easily in the front and were not open down the back. Treatment required no extra baring of flesh. The shirts had a name, too, a good one: dignity robes.

Dignity: Intrinsic worth, also, gravity and poise. Can a shirt do all that? In this case, yes, because the shirt was all of a piece with the clinic. At RadOnc they cared. They cared about the big things, like making sure I understood how my treatment would go, and the little things, like feeling bad about not having Aquaphor on hand to give away. So bring on the dignity robes, with their pseudo-psychedelic patterns on thick, mud-brown cloth. Bring on the video, which has gotten mixed up in my mind with the videos they show on airplanes before take-off: "Here are the safety features of our airplane" versus "Here are the cancer-fighting features of radiation oncology." Bring on the radiologist, who was clear and efficiently reassuring. Bring on the waiting room that had a Keurig machine and a way to make hot tea, and a receptionist who said "Oh, it doesn't matter" if I forgot to sign in electronically with my right index finger on the stand-alone computer located right across from her desk.

Nothing can make a cancer diagnosis better. There is bad and worse. There's also terrible. And there's tragic. What I wanted, and what I got in radiation oncology, was the feeling that people cared enough to make treatment *easier*. Right down to letting me sit in the hallway outside the waiting room, because watching snippets of game shows and commercials on the waiting room TV made me, for reasons I cannot figure out, anxious. Five days a week for four weeks, a friendly technician stepped out into the hallway and called me in for each of my appointments, without ever implying that I was putting them out.

Forgetfulness hit me like an extra symptom of cancer once I was diagnosed; trauma theorists assert that forgetting and rearranging memories are common for trauma victims. Did having cancer make me a trauma victim? Me, with my stage-1, found-on-ultrasound breast cancer. Well, of course. What a surprise, then, that I actually have some pretty great memories from RadOnc, and despite the large, pricey machines and the sci-fi vibe of the place, it was old-fashioned concern and basic politeness that made my radiation treatments *feel* better than other aspects of my cancer care.

So, here's my question. If they can be compassionate at radiation oncology, why can't they be that way everywhere else?

TWENTY

Slow Burn

PEOPLE HAD TOLD me radiation would make me tired. I'd also heard stories about patients getting terrible burns from the treatments, but those were from years ago, before radiation oncologists learned that smaller, targeted doses prevented disease recurrence just as well as much larger ones.

The techs had drawn crosses on my chest to aim the beams, and I worried the crosses would come off from sweating during my bike rides to and from treatment. They reassured me that the crosses could be reapplied as often as needed. They had also created a mold of my body that would help make me more comfortable and minimize movement during treatment. I lay down on the mold on the narrow table, the techs adjusted the beams of radiation, and the drum of the big machine rotated around me. The process itself took about ten minutes. I brought my ugly shirt every day and every day I changed into and out of it, before and after treatment, in one of the two small dressing rooms set off from the main treatment hallway. The techs were always, or nearly always, right on time.

Except for the two mornings each week that I worked out, I made no plans for before or after treatment. If I had planned to get together with a friend and ended up being too tired, I would have had to cancel, and I didn't want to have to apologize to anyone.

Treatment was at eleven a.m., I think. That was my time. *Let's Make a Deal* was always wrapping up on the TV when I checked in. Was anyone ever offered a deal to have her cancer go away? I sat out in the hallway and worked on the *New York Times* crossword puzzle. Sometimes I read a book, occasionally a magazine I brought with me. The maternity department was located kitty-corner to RadOnc and I watched couples go in together, the women's bellies swollen, the men hovering attentively. I studied the geometric pattern of the carpet and listened to the player piano in the hospital's first-floor atrium. The machines used for radiation treatments are heavy, so RadOnc departments are often in hospital basements. This department was no exception, but the comfortable chairs in the hallway were a cheerful cherry red and I enjoyed watching patients, staff, housekeepers, and maintenance workers come and go.

My goal had been to ride my bike to and from treatment at least four out of the five days of treatment the whole four weeks, and I did. I was not trying to prove that I'm tougher than cancer, not exactly. I am not Lance Armstrong, obviously, who we now know is a doper and a liar anyway. His book is called *It's Not About the Bike*, but for me it kind of was, because riding my bike to and from treatment made me feel alive. The idea of driving to the hospital every day, parking, getting treated, leaving the parking lot when I was done, and driving home again, made me feel depressed before I even started. I rode to prove to myself that my body was not broken. I rode my bike because I needed to.

The first week of radiation, the sun shone and I didn't need my snow pants or even winter gloves. I zigzagged through streets in the neighborhood and went down a hill, praying to make the light at the bottom so that I could sail through the intersection and get halfway up the next small hill without pedaling. I got to Pittsburgh's Schenley Park, the absolute best part of the ride, where a long, slow uphill led to a downhill just steep enough to send me shooting, free, down to the main road to the hospital. The wind hit my face hard as I flew into it, but that first week was unusually warm for December; it didn't hurt.

People say it's not the destination, it's the journey. Yeah, right. If you're going to radiation therapy, it's the destination. When I got to the hospital, I locked my bike to the world's loneliest-looking bike rack, planted in the middle of a slab of concrete, surrounded by black metal fencing. It offered no shade from the sun or shield from rain or snow, and my bike was often the only one there.

The next day of treatment was the same, and the next day and the next, except all the downhills were uphills on the return ride. Once on the way home, as I rode through the U. Pitt neighborhood, I saw my daughter Sophia walking to class. I called out and she and I smiled and waved at each other. I occasionally stopped at our local corner grocery store and bought a turkey sandwich for lunch. Other times I made myself a perfect poached egg and toast after I got to the house. If it was very cold, I would make hot chocolate.

The second week of treatment the winter cold struck, and I wanted a new way home with fewer cars. My usual ride home involved a long uphill with steady traffic and multiple cars parked along the route selling food out of their trunks to students—lunchtime. I didn't like riding up that hill with all the cars and Arthur suggested that I ride back through Schenley Park, taking a different route than I rode to get to treatment, up the slow, steep hill that wound through the park's public golf course. It would be longer than my old route and slightly harder, but it was better. There were many fewer cars, and I had enticing green on both sides at the steepest part.

I did that ride in rain so hard it blurred my vision through my glasses and I did it with sleet pinging painfully against my unprotected cheeks and freezing my hands inside my Gore-Tex lined gloves. I did it on a few unexpectedly warm days on which golfers appeared out on the green, rolling their big bags of clubs behind them, and I wondered, vaguely, if I risked being hit in the head with a ball. I rode past people walking up the hill and I waved to people zipping down the alternate side on bikes of their own.

That second week when it was so cold, I made hot tea when I got to the radiation treatment center. "How does it feel to ride your bike in this weather?" the receptionist asked, her brow furrowed with curiosity and concern.

"Well, it's pretty cold," I said, and she nodded.

The next day, one of the techs asked how I managed with icy sleet hitting my face. "Lots of moisturizer," I said, my fingers still so cold I couldn't completely feel them.

On the third day of below-freezing temperatures, I drove to my appointment because it was really snowing and it was just too cold. "You're still my hero," one of the techs told me.

A word about the radiation techs, who were incredible human beings, always friendly and professional. "We know you don't want to be here so it's extra important for us to be nice," one of them explained. They were all so young, in their twenties, and yet they demonstrated something so important about people, about healing. They knew the value of kindness. If the sole intention of this book was to laud the people who best recognized my humanity during my cancer treatment, it would focus on the techs in RadOnc. Halfway through the treatment they offered me permanent tattoos to replace the drawn-on crosses on my skin that they kept having to redraw because sweat from bike riding would fade them. The tattoos take only a few minutes to place and the first one went on my sternum. I don't remember feeling it, but one of the techs said, "Wow. Most people really flinch at that one. It hurts. You just took it, stone cold."

"Stone cold," I said. "I like that." Seems like I did want to be tougher than cancer. I still have the tattoos—little blue dots—and will have them forever. A reminder, like the scar on my right breast.

The last day of treatment, Arthur and I took lunch to the techs. There was a deli nearby and I bought a ridiculous amount of food for the three or four of them who might be working. I hoped that a real lunch would be a treat and that they would have time to eat the large sandwiches, big enough for two people, put their feet up and bite into one of the crisp apples. Afterwards they could lick melted chocolate from the oversized cookies off their fingers, along with traces of salt from the potato chips.

Every Monday I saw the radiation oncologist. She checked my skin and made sure that, in general, I was doing OK. The Monday of the fourth and last week, I couldn't stop crying as I waited for her. Over the weekend I had that sudden spell of inconsolable crying, too, when I walked alone in Frick Park. I told the doctor that I felt afraid of dying and asked, "Am I losing it?"

"No," she said, shaking her head. Turns out, most people are able to put their fear aside during treatment because the schedule pulls them along and makes them feel they are *doing something to fight the disease*. When treatment nears its end and patients anticipate living their regular lives still bearing the emotional and physical weight of having had cancer, the fear returns. "You're right on schedule," she told me.

This was comforting. The thought of my own death really scared me, but many patients felt similarly frightened at the same point in radiation therapy. Fear was normal. And soon my treatment would be over and my cancer would not have killed me. I had more time to live and I would keep on living. In other words, I was right on schedule.

TWENTY-ONE

Pickles

ANYONE EXPECTING THIS chapter to be a paean to bread-and-butter slices, sour dills, cornichons, gherkins, the English Ploughman's, or Branstons will be disappointed. This chapter does not discuss cravings that radiation treatment caused, or foods I ate to soothe myself when the worry felt like too much. This chapter is about our dog, named Pickles.

My medical oncologist, Dr. Y, was forthright and clear, but she was not warm and fuzzy. I knew that when I chose her, same as I knew it about my surgeon. As a nurse, I'd had patients whose doctors lied to them, mentally fortified them with half-truths and false hope, and some of those patients ended up dying very ugly deaths because their actual prognosis had been withheld. I wanted what I thought of as *the truth* from my physicians: technical detail combined with explanations I understood, along with accurate information about treatment risks and benefits. Dr. Y and Dr. S did all that beautifully. But part of me still longed for warmth and kindness, same as when

I regretted not choosing the surgeon who would have held my hand and said, "You are going to be OK."

I came to see that I did get the sympathetic care I wanted—from my dog. A dog is literally warm and fuzzy, and some afternoons, after radiation, I would lie down on our living room couch for a nap, and Pickles would jump up and lie down on top of me. She's about forty-five pounds and I found her bulk soothing. Pickles, named after a dog in an odd but much-loved children's book, Beatrix Potter's *Ginger and Pickles*, was a great comfort to me.

I'm not trying to make an exhaustive claim about dogs or people's relationships with their dogs in this brief chapter. I want to say something about recognizing comfort where we find it. My dog could not tell me, *You will be OK*, because, of course, she is a dog. She knows nothing about the ins and outs of breast cancer diagnoses and treatments. She recognizes pain, though, and vulnerability, and she cared for me in a primal way, with her body, her warmth, her undeniable doggy *thereness*. I admit now that I wanted more from my oncologist and my surgeon: empathy, compassion, and solace. Pickles offered all three in her way. Her weight on me made me feel like being held—being held together, almost.

TWENTY-TWO

A Friend in Need

MATTHEW JOHNSON WAS my husband's colleague in the University of Pittsburgh Physics Department. They also played music together, my husband on piano, Matthew on clarinet. Matthew had a twinkle in his eye, a distinctive laugh that came easily, and a mischievous smile. That might sound unusual for a physicist, but it describes him. And one day I showed up at the hospital and he was my patient.

I'm writing in the past tense, but Matthew is still very much alive. He belongs to our, and more important, his own, present, although he's retired from teaching physics. Matthew had colon cancer, which for most people gets treated out-patient, meaning no hospital stays. His chemo, though, had made him sick enough that he needed to be hospitalized.

That day I worked the evening shift: from three in the afternoon until eleven p.m. It's a shift no one likes because it doesn't have any kind of natural rhythm. I didn't know how caring for Matthew would go. Perhaps he would rather not have his colleague's wife be his nurse, I thought, worried about his dignity and privacy, but those were not his concerns. When I started the shift, his problem was pain.

I entered his room tentatively, ready to give a short speech about how he could have a different nurse if he preferred. But he didn't seem to recognize me. His features were fixed in a grimace, his eyes squinting, and his whole body had turned in on itself as he sat up in the bed, shoulders hunched forward, arms guarding his belly. He was still and afraid to move and I will never forget the look on his face. Using bits and pieces of sentences, he made it clear that he had asked for pain medication a while ago and hadn't gotten it. I had seen a lot of people suffer in the hospital, but not like that. Or maybe, not people I knew.

My carefully prepared remarks on the appropriateness of being Matthew's nurse went unsaid. Instead, I hurried out of the room, down the hallway to the locked room where we kept the narcotics inside a locked machine. I entered the passcode, typed Matthew's name, and waited until the correct drawer and lid popped open. I took out one vial, counted the rest and punched the number of remaining vials back into the computer, closed the lid and pushed the drawer back in. *Hurry, hurry, hurry,* I told myself as I went briskly back up the hallway.

At my medication cart, I drew the narcotic up into a syringe, diluted it in saline, and went into the room to give it to Matthew through his IV. He barely acknowledged me being there and I started to worry that pain was not his only issue, that something could be clouding his mind. This happened while I was still on the floor with the bullies, where keeping to myself was the safest bet, so I didn't ask anyone how Matthew had been doing, and I didn't report the nurse who had him before me and left him to suffer.

The drug usually kicked in in fifteen to thirty minutes. "Stay ahead of the pain," we say, as if it's a train you need to outrun. Matthew's pain got the better of him because it got past us. *We* failed him, but *he* suffered.

That night at the hospital, I talked on the phone with a family friend of Matthew's who was a physician. She wanted to piece together what exactly had happened to Matthew medically. Matthew himself had complained to me, once his pain was under control, that in his view most MDs weren't good at thinking. Physicists were good at thinking, he said, but not many doctors, and he needed the people taking care of him to think about what had gone wrong with him. I did the best I could with Matthew's friend's questions, but what I remember most was her saying that when the family heard I had been assigned as Matthew's nurse they had described that as "a good thing."

A few days later I returned to work and saw Matthew in the hospital as he walked the halls wearing a fleecy, oversized burgundy robe. It made him look like a king, but of a kingdom where the royalty all dressed like teddy bears. His wife, Linda, was with him and the twinkle had returned to his eyes. He was going home the next day.

LATER, LITERALLY YEARS later, after my own diagnosis, Matthew invited Arthur and me over to dinner. Well, to be honest, I think Linda masterminded the invitation and the meal, but no matter. I was in the middle of radiation treatments and my thinking was so fuzzy it felt like my brain had been replaced with cotton balls.

After a dinner of perfectly roasted chicken and herbed green beans, Matthew told me he never thinks about cancer anymore. He lives in its shadow only every now and then, when he has a checkup or a scan. I'd seen him over the years, of course, playing music with Arthur, or at a party we threw, or at his own retirement party. I would always give him a big hug and then earnestly ask how he was, until I realized he didn't need me to ask anymore, or at least not like that.

One afternoon in the hospital, I took care of Matthew when he had been neglected. Over a decade later, when I needed it, he returned the favor with his story: that there is life after cancer.

TWENTY-THREE

Spatchcock

RADIATION ENDED RIGHT before Christmas. I threw away my ugly, beloved dignity gown. I put it in a plastic bag before I put it in our garbage can, as if it were toxic and I didn't want the poison to leak out. Truth is, I wanted to burn it, to obliterate it into ash, which is what I wanted for my whole breast cancer experience. I wanted any remnants of treatment gone.

It was a few days before Christmas. I had suggested we do family gifts. Whoever wanted to get presents for others could, but the presents needed to be for all of us collectively. The three kids bought a large, intricate board game called Immortals, which was a half-serious, half-joking present. They love board games and decided to buy the most complicated game they could find. Then they played it with Arthur over the break. I lay on the couch in our sunroom and read a murder mystery while they sat around the table, learning the game as they played. The background noise consisted of them discussing the rules, murmuring over cards, asking what was supposed to happen next, and trying to figure out how the game ended. The game parts included a small tower made out of cardboard, and at intervals, dice representing armies went into the top of the tower and rolled out the bottom, interjecting randomness into a game that seemed confusing enough already. It took them two nights to finish one go-round.

For Christmas dinner, my son ordered quail from one of the stores in Pittsburgh's Strip District, a collection of restaurants, bakeries, coffee places, and butcher shops. A former vegetarian, Conrad thinks that quails are "cute." When he unwrapped the quails, though, he was disappointed and annoyed to see that the store had partially deboned and then flattened each bird, leaving in only their wings and leg bones to give the remainder of the bird some structure. Conrad is an inventive cook. The quail he had imagined roasting still had all their bones.

Readying quail, or any fowl like this, followed by grilling, has a peculiar name: spatchcock. It can be a noun—a bird split and cooked—or a verb, which means to prepare a bird in that way. Spatchcocking a quail requires slicing down its back to remove the backbone, because with the backbone gone, the quail can be easily flattened. I wondered why they spatch-cocked the quail when Conrad had not asked for that. Maybe our order got mixed up with someone else's, who was now unhappy about receiving bony quail for Christmas. Or perhaps at that store quail always came that way unless the customer requested otherwise.

The problem was, if Conrad cares about something, he cares about it a lot. He wanted the quail to have backbones and he energetically told me why the backbones mattered. As

I listened, he grew calmer, and got a new idea, a variation on his original plan. He baked the spatchcocked quail covered in olive oil, freshly ground black pepper, and a shower of rosemary leaves. *Oh my goodness.* The quail tasted so good the meal felt like a gift.

Christmas has always been my favorite holiday, with the story of Mary and Joseph and the birth of Jesus in a manger, surrounded by cows and sheep, visited afterwards by shepherds and the Magi as they are celebrated in song. I also like the twinkling of Christmas lights, the sharp smell of pine, the crinkling of wrapping paper, and having enough snow for an actual white Christmas. That Christmas, though, coming so soon after the end of radiation, I felt spatchcocked. The kids decorated the tree and Conrad organized the meals since I felt useless, as if my backbone had been removed and I had been flattened down.

It wasn't that I couldn't enjoy Christmas, I just couldn't experience it as I usually did. I didn't feel much of anything except bewilderment, fatigue, and a strong urge to be done with cancer, to turn the corner on my diagnosis and disease by moving into the new year. I was already so over it, or wanted to be, but it's not that simple. Once cancer comes, it hangs around in your mind, whether welcome or not. It can ruin holidays, anniversaries, planned vacations, retirements, years of people's lives. Some would say that because my active treatment lasted only a few months, I got off easy. I kind of understand what those people mean, but they have failed to grasp how having cancer can feel.

If only I could have removed my fear as easily as the butcher removed the backbones from all those quail. If only forgetting was as straightforward as picking up a small dead bird and flattening it, wings included, never minding that its tiny, cold heart was left vulnerable and exposed.

PART THREE

Out of the Frying Pan

TWENTY-FOUR

Tam

MY DAD USED to wear tams. He had two and they suited him. The hat of Scotsmen, with that flat wide crown and sometimes a pompom in the middle, except never on my dad's tams. His father was a carpenter from small-town Missouri who never attended college, and yet my dad became a philosophy professor. His PhD seems like an off-scale achievement considering his background. No wonder then, with his bushy mustache and dark hair swept back from his forehead, with his ceramic mugs of coffee that steamed and spilled as he carried them out to the car on cold winter mornings, no wonder he could carry off a tam.

Me, my version of tam, it didn't go nearly as well. But then again, for a lot of women it doesn't. I started Tamoxifen on January first—the beginning of the new year. My medical oncologist suggested I make January 1 my start date since I'd finished radiation a week and a half earlier and that date would make it easy to remember when I started. She was right.

My mom took Tamoxifen for five years as a preventive for breast cancer. She had no problems with the drug, but then again, she never has problems with any medications. Except for having hairy cell leukemia in middle age, my mom has the strongest constitution of anyone I know. I might have thought that the ease with which my mother adjusted to Tamoxifen was unusual if I had known more about it, but I rarely worked with breast cancer patients as a nurse, and when I did, it was always with patients whose disease had proved stronger than the available treatment. So, I thought that being on Tamoxifen would be fine. "I'll take it for five years," I would say, as if announcing some wonderful new habit I planned to pick up, like becoming a vegetarian, or walking strenuously in the early morning five days a week.

However, my mom was done with menopause when she took Tamoxifen, and I wasn't quite. That was one difference. My mom had also never been plagued with irregular periods or had menstrual cramps so painful and nauseating they sent her to bed. I had, and that was another difference. Women with breast cancer get put on Tamoxifen because their tumor is estrogen-receptor positive. Some women gain weight and some have their hair fall out. Others have such a high degree of confusion—called "brain fog"—that they feel they must choose between quitting their jobs or quitting Tamoxifen. Some have hot flashes so severe that they can't sleep, and they can't take estrogen to control the hot flashes because estrogen will stimulate the growth of cancer cells if the patient has a recurrence of disease.

Tamoxifen is a dirty drug. I take it because I can't imagine not doing that and then explaining to my kids why I relapsed.

The odds of that happening are small, but I refuse to accept the risk. The day after I started it, my period started, very much out of sync. I wondered if this was the bleeding risk that came with the drug. A noted side effect of Tamoxifen is vaginal hemorrhage. Another side effect is blood clots. I wasn't hemorrhaging or clotting, as far as I could tell, but I called the doctor's office anyway, because I felt chilled, too—chilled to the bone. They wanted me to take my temperature to make sure I didn't have a fever. "I don't have a fever. I'm a nurse," I said, as if the two things were naturally related, but they wanted me to check, so I did. My temperature was normal, unlike having my period start *just like that*, but the nurse didn't find it worrisome.

A few days later I woke up with the worst headache I have ever had. I briefly suffered from migraines when I took birth-control pills. Those were bad, but if I stayed horizontal as much as possible when I had one, it would pass. This headache was different. Sharp pain spread over the entire crown of my head, concentrated almost in a line straight down the middle of my forehead, from my hairline to the bridge of my nose. It felt like someone had bisected my forehead with an axe. The pain was so intense it seemed to be alive. I couldn't escape it and I couldn't medicate it away, though I tried with over-the-counter pain medicine. Terrible nausea and a revulsion to all food accompanied the pain. I stayed in bed. I didn't have much choice.

In *Into Thin Air*, Jon Krakauer's account of his attempt to scale Mount Everest, Krakauer writes about how, after reaching the summit and contending with a horrific winter storm, he huddled in his tent, too depleted to do anything but lie there.

He felt physically unable to help his fellow climbers, some of whom were dying in the cold and snow. When I have had the flu, before I understood the wisdom of getting a flu shot, I felt that way—so played out that I could do nothing besides stay in bed, hoping for the fever, chills, and body aches to pass. This headache from Tamoxifen felt the same.

Tamoxifen is in a class of drugs known as SERMs, selective estrogen receptor modulators. Don't know what that is? Let's check UpToDate, an online database of medications that health care professionals use:

> Tamoxifen is a selective estrogen receptor modulator (SERM) that competitively binds to estrogen receptors on tumors and other tissue targets, producing a nuclear complex that decreases DNA synthesis and inhibits estrogen effects; nonsteroidal agent with potent anti-estrogenic properties which compete with estrogen for binding sites in breast and other tissues; cells accumulate in the G_0 and G_1 phases; therefore, tamoxifen is cytostatic rather than cytocidal.

As a patient once said to me after her medical team talked to her in the hospital, "Well, that was clear as mud, wasn't it?" The human body is made up of different kinds of tissue: muscle, nerve, brain, bone, and so on. Every tissue type consists of cells unique to that tissue, and each cell has receptors that can be activated to provoke or inhibit a bodily response: I bend my arm when my brain sends an electrical impulse to the muscles of my arm, signaling them to contract. We have receptors

throughout our bodies for pain and pain relief, to enable diges-
tion, to make medications work, and for hormones. My breast
cancer had growth receptors for estrogen, and estrogen is the
primary female sex hormone. That's a problem. Tamoxifen
keeps estrogen from binding to estrogen receptors by "com-
petitively" binding with those receptors instead. As UpToDate
explains, Tamoxifen keeps estrogen away from the tumor.

The "G_0 and G_1 phases" are the first and second stages of a
cell's typical growth cycle. The cell rests in G_0. In G_1, the cell
becomes larger, preparing for division—reproduction, really,
since cells reproduce by dividing—but Tamoxifen arrests cellular development in either G_0 or G_1 and cells that cannot advance
past G_1 cannot reproduce. If, after surgery and radiation, my
body contained any remaining cancer cells, Tamoxifen should
prevent those cells from dividing and over time becoming a
malignant mass. Because it doesn't kill cancer cells, Tamoxifen
isn't cytocidal, but cytostatic, meaning it renders malignant
cells ineffectual by inhibiting their growth. Solid tumor cancers occur because normal brakes on cellular growth have gone
haywire. Tamoxifen keeps potentially malignant cells, those
with broken brakes, in stasis, or at least that's the idea.

Also, Tamoxifen gets the job done. Different studies show
that it lowers the risk of a breast cancer recurrence by 30, 40,
even 50 percent. In every study I examined, Tamoxifen lowered
recurrence rates to a statistically significant degree, and I was
unable to find any studies showing otherwise. But let's consider that risk reduction more fully. A 2017 article in the *New
England Journal of Medicine* puts my risk of recurrence at 10
percent within twenty years (the article is specific for my type

of breast cancer, among others). If Tamoxifen cuts my recurrence risk by 30 percent—the value given in the article—then I go from an overall 10 percent risk of recurrence to a 7 percent risk. That matters, but of course, what I really want is a drug that lowers my recurrence risk to 0 percent, that eliminates any risk of recurrence. I want a drug that says, in bold, on the bottle: **Take this medicine and you will never get cancer again.**

TWENTY-FIVE

Tam, Continued

SOME STUDIES ESTIMATE that half of all women with ER+ breast cancer who are prescribed Tamoxifen discontinue it before the recommended five years are up. And there are also women who refuse to start the drug at all. As a friend from the publishing industry told me via email, explaining her decision never to begin Tamoxifen, "I need my brain."

I need my brain, too, but I made a different choice. Audre Lorde, in her autobiographical book *The Cancer Journals*, writes, "Each woman responds to the crisis that breast cancer brings to her life out of a whole pattern, which is the design of who she is and how her life has been lived. The weave of her every day existence is the training ground for how she handles crisis." I believe this. I told my friend that each woman makes the best decision she can for herself alone. I don't judge. She could just as easily judge me, a writer, for staying on Tamoxifen, willingly tamping down my intellect for a drug that reduces my risk of recurrence, but doesn't eliminate it.

Women quit Tamoxifen because their hair falls out. Others quit because they gain weight and some because they become depressed. Another cohort of Tamoxifen rebels can't take the nighttime hot flashes the drug causes along with the accompanying insomnia. For others, it's the fatigue, and for women like my friend in publishing, and a friend of a friend, the brain fog is intolerable. I have had hot flashes, fatigue, and brain fog. The hot flashes were irksome, but not deal breakers, though in addition to the hot flashes, or as a result of the hot flashes, if I overheat, I now sweat profusely. Walking even a short distance on a warm day will leave a sheen of sweat on the back of my neck and rivulets of sweat will run down my back. If I go for a walk when it's hot out, I will finish looking like I sat in a sauna fully dressed.

The sweating is annoying, but the fatigue and brain fog have been harder to manage. Both were intense when I started Tamoxifen. I had planned to return to hospice nursing that January since I had finished active treatment, but a return to work was not possible considering how tired and mentally slow I often felt. If Arthur and I had needed my income, or if I had wanted to work as a way to restart my normal life, I would probably have gone off Tamoxifen. That's no kind of a choice for a cancer patient to have to make.

Some women need a three-month adjustment period when starting birth control pills. I always did, and on that basis, I decided to give myself three months to adjust to Tamoxifen. It was a long three months. In late February I took my daughter Miranda and a teammate of hers to Chapel Hill, North

Carolina, to try out for the American Women's World's Team in Ultimate Frisbee. I had a hard time following the directions my daughter gave me for driving the rental car from the airport to our hotel. Once we got there and settled in, though, my confusion began to really clear for the first time.

I had an article due and I wrote it while Miranda and her friend were at tryouts during the day. I drove them to and from the practice fields and picked out restaurants I thought they would like for dinner and drove us to those meals. My concentration had returned, but I had no idea why. Was it being in a new place? The strong coffee I bought at a nearby coffeeshop? The mental work of putting together an essay? I doubt it was the ambiance of our cheap motel, where the large glass windows in our room that looked out at the too-cold-to-swim-in pool stayed permanently clouded due to the mist that fell all weekend.

That March, over the university's spring break, and still within my three-month adjustment period, Arthur, Miranda, Sophia, and I went to Harper's Ferry, West Virginia, to hike for a few days. My confusion was better, but tiredness enveloped me like the end-of-winter chill on the Appalachian Trail. We hiked—eight miles one day, ten the next—returning at night to our charming one-bedroom cottage with a small kitchen and a loft bed for the twins. I did both hikes and I kept up. Mostly. If I felt tired on an uphill, I had to stop. I didn't feel short of breath or out of shape, but like I had stalled and revving the engine would not help. I felt frustrated at the drug, at myself, but I was also too tired to be agitated. *This is not me*, I wanted to say. And yet undeniably it was me feeling so much fatigue on those hikes in Harper's Ferry.

Spatchcock. This time it felt like I lost my muscles, not my bones, but it's the same idea. I could not make myself go faster and at the end of each day, I had to lie down while Arthur made dinner in the small kitchen. I had planned our meals but could not prepare them myself. I wanted to scream at the world, but the world wasn't listening. I wanted energy, drive, ambition, and I couldn't find it anywhere inside me. It had, simply, gone. *I'm a type A person whom medication turned into a type B person.* This is what I told myself. And it's not a bad thing to have to slow down. I tried to believe that.

On our two hikes, we saw austerely beautiful patches of forest, groves of trees stuck in the deadness of late winter, their bare branches reaching beseechingly to the sky. We walked along the Potomac, its icy waters hurtling along, gathering force for spring. All I could think was, *When will this hike end?*

I would like to say the beauty of the scenery soothed me.

I would like to say that being in nature restored me.

I would like to say that having this wonderful time with my husband and daughters was enough. Because it was a wonderful time. But it wasn't enough.

I'm living the trade-off. I'm living with what cancer, and cancer treatment, took away from me. And I mind, an awful lot actually.

I am still alive and of course I would rather be alive and tired than dead. But gratitude for my life does not lessen my tiredness or, despite how mentally sharp I felt in Chapel Hill, my ongoing intermittent confusion. I can bear quite a bit, but it feels like Tam aged me before my time. Some might argue that that is not a high price to pay for my life and they would be right, are right. But their being right doesn't help me. Is it so hard to see that both things can be true?

TWENTY-SIX

Tam, Conclusion

I FELT MORE normal once I'd been on Tamoxifen for three months, and once again gave talks, worked on this book, and went back to work in hospice after being away for about half a year (more on that later). Those are not humble-brags. The point is, Tamoxifen messed with my sense of competence. The drug changed my perception of who I was, and yet, on the surface, I mostly remained the same. I did all the same stuff I had done before, only everything took a little more effort than it had. I could no longer rely on my spectacular memory and ability to focus intently on details. I felt mentally dull.

People told me that my symptoms sounded a lot like normal aging, that, "It only gets worse." But unless I somehow aged very rapidly the day I started taking Tamoxifen, my exhaustion and confusion weren't a result of getting older. Some days I felt fairly close to normal, and then suddenly I would have to lie down and sleep for three to four extra hours to be functional. That challenged my Protestant work ethic and chipped away at my self-esteem. For the first time in my life, at my worst moments, and even though I knew better, I saw myself as lazy.

NOW WE JUMP ahead. After two years of taking Tamoxifen, almost to the date, I started to really feel like myself again. The return to normal accompanied a kind of accidental decision to stop taking vitamin D, which I'd started during radiation treatments because my Vitamin D level was low. Curious, I did research on possible connections between Tam and vitamin D, but nothing I read applied to my set of symptoms. Still, I blamed vitamin D for the worst of my symptoms. *It wasn't Tamoxifen at all*, I thought wryly.

Fast forward almost three years. My parathyroid level is slightly elevated. The surgical endocrinologist I see tells me that the most common reason for such elevations is a low level of vitamin D. She prescribes a fairly high dose of vitamin D combined with calcium in response, and when my parathyroid hormone level trends down, but is still high, and my vitamin D level is still low, she increases the dose of vitamin D. How do I feel? The same, for a while. The fatigue and brain fog do not come back. But after a few months of high doses of vitamin D, I start to have terrible insomnia and terrible exhaustion. I feel like I can't think at all. Worst of all, the hot flashes I have when trying to fall asleep, or when sleeping, are so terrible I wake up. Sweat covers my torso during the night and my pajamas are soaked in the morning.

I complain about this sudden onset of much worse symptoms to Arthur and he asks, "Aren't you taking a high dose of vitamin D again?" Bingo. The symptoms came back just different enough that I failed to put the pieces together. I stopped taking extra vitamin D and informed the endocrinologist. The brain fog, insomnia, exhaustion, and terrible hot flashes all went away. I still take the combined calcium and vitamin D with no issues beyond what is typical for me with Tamoxifen, and my parathyroid level returned to normal once my calcium and vitamin D levels did, too. The endocrinologist could not explain my negative response to the higher level of vitamin D, though she had seen it before. She said that people usually do better with vitamin D combined with calcium in one pill, and that supplement has been fine for me.

I appreciated her honesty and that she believed me when I described my strange symptoms. I have a similarly idiosyncratic response to Benadryl, the antihistamine known by the generic name diphenhydramine. Twice I was prescribed Benadryl for hives and twice it made my body explode with hives and my arms swell up like overinflated balloons. I have told different doctors this story and one agreed that Benadryl had made my hives worse, and one put the whole thing down to "coincidence." But I won't take Benadryl if I'm having an allergic reaction and I threw away the extra vitamin D I had on hand. Don't go back to a dog that bites expecting a different dog.

TWENTY-SEVEN

On the Side

CONSIDER ONE HOSPITAL patient, back when I worked on the bone-marrow transplant floor. I went into his room to administer scheduled chemo, and he asked a simple question, "Will this make my neuropathy worse?" Will this make the tingling, numbness, and pain in my feet worse, he wanted to know. The answer was, maybe. About 30 to 40 percent of patients who receive chemo get peripheral neuropathy in their hands and/or feet. The problem is common enough that it has its own acronym: CIPN, for chemotherapy-induced peripheral neuropathy.

Certain drugs cause it, but not for everyone, and certain drugs don't. Whether a person already has neuropathies, from diabetes, for example, can factor hugely into whether chemo makes them worse. With this patient, I split the difference. "It can cause neuropathy," I said, giving an answer pretty much guaranteed to satisfy no one.

He got mad so quickly that it surprised me. "Well, that's going to make the neuropathy even worse!" he spit out. Some leukemia patients had such intense neuropathy in their feet that they could barely walk, either because the pain couldn't be managed or because they no longer felt their feet well enough to balance. This is normal. Normal. And it's a terrible devil's bargain, too.

This patient was the first to crack my clinical ethical certainties, my surety that we hurt people for their own good, that the trade-off was worth it because *we saved their lives*. Of course. *Of course*. But in the meantime, his feet hurt and walking was hard and I, we, did that to him. We cured him and we crippled him. Not a metaphor but a fact. His losing his temper surprised me because it was so rare. Our patients had complaints, but in general they came across as grateful, not irate. If they were angry, they directed acrimony at their disease, at being stuck in the hospital, at the financial cost of their care, at having to go to the bathroom and having to try to sleep attached to an IV pump that sometimes would not stop beeping. They expressed rage at the unfairness of it all. This patient, though, was upset about his treatment and he let me know it. His gratitude for being alive did not mitigate the pain in his feet and I felt like an idiot for imagining that it would.

A different patient. This man had a new diagnosis of leukemia, like Bob of Bob and Wendy. He was hospitalized for a minimum six weeks of induction chemotherapy, and I was often his nurse. He ran his own business as a wholesale supplier and, before he got leukemia, worked constantly. His diagnosis meant he had to stay in the hospital and essentially do nothing for longer than he ever had in his adult life. The change in circumstances was hard for him, and as time passed, he seemed to grow increasingly depressed. He kept the lights in his room turned off and the blinds drawn, twenty-four hours a day. I suggested he talk to a therapist, try taking an antidepressant. He refused both.

He had pain in his right rear hipbone, the site of a bone-marrow biopsy, a procedure that extracts actual bone marrow by drilling into the hip with a hand-held tool. Patients sometimes had pain in that spot for a few days after a biopsy, though some had little pain during the procedure or after. But this patient's pain would not go away: sharp, stabbing, it radiated out from the site of the biopsy, making him miserable.

None of his doctors could explain his pain, so, I'm sorry to say, they ignored it and subtly implied that he wasn't really in pain or that the pain wasn't as bad as he said. This is a problem in modern health care—what can't be explained sometimes gets denied as real. The thinking seemed to be that since no one ever had pain like his so long after a bone-marrow biopsy, this patient shouldn't, or couldn't, be having that pain either. I listened to him, talked with his doctors, argued for better pain management for him, but nothing I, or anyone else, did really helped. After having been his nurse for so long, I was cycled away from him to other patients and only got updates when I asked. Then he was gone.

One day, months later, I was at work and suddenly he appeared in front of me, a new man. For one thing, he smiled. His arms hung loosely at his sides and his hands were open, relaxed, as he bent towards me and we hugged hello.

I asked how he'd been feeling, about his work, the business. "Oh, I only work when I feel like it," he said. He smiled again and I swear I saw a twinkle in his eye. As he spoke, he pushed his palms together in front of him, like he was flattening his former obsession with work. "When I get tired, I stop," he said. I have thought about this patient so often. For me, he represented proof of concept. We put people through the ringer, but in the end, their treatment changed them for the better. *We saved their lives and changed them for the better.*

This is the note I wish I could end on. As a nurse I struggled when patients had difficult side effects, but in the end, as this patient ably demonstrated, patients in general benefited from our care and were happy to have received it. But *I* am now a patient and I don't feel that way. Or rather, I do, and I don't.

Fatigue, it turns out, is the number one symptom that afflicts cancer patients, including after they have finished treatment, necessitating yet another acronym: CRF for cancer-related fatigue. Oncologists are researching it, taking it seriously despite their inability to explain it. The National Comprehensive Cancer Network (NCCN) defines CRF as "a distressing persistent, subjective sense of physical, emotional and/or cognitive tiredness related to cancer or cancer treatment that is not proportional to recent activity and interferes with usual functioning."

One theory, proposed by Julienne Bower et al. holds that CRF is caused by genetic sequences that promote inflammation, the process that gives us a runny nose when we have a cold, or makes injuries get red and swell. Their research found that breast cancer patients with genetic variants that stimulate, or perhaps overstimulate, the body's inflammatory response have the greatest level of fatigue. A different paper, by César

Fernández-de-las-Peñas et al., explored the link between a gene sequence named COMT and postcancer levels of pain and fatigue in breast cancer patients. They describe their work as a breakthrough because it establishes that high degrees of pain and fatigue may result from genetic factors unique to individual patients: "These results are innovative in that they represent the first evidence of a link between a risk factor for cancer-related fatigue, increased pain sensitivity, and COMT genotype in breast cancer."

The science is fascinating, although ultimately unhelpful to patients, including me, right now. I wonder if my health insurance would have paid for genetic sequencing to see if I had the pro-fatigue genes, but even if it did, and I do, it's not clear that knowing that would do me any practical good. I was very fatigued, which I attributed to Tamoxifen, but maybe it resulted from radiation, or the cancer, or vitamin D, or my own genetic make-up, or some combination of all five. Regardless of what triggered the fatigue, I found it very difficult.

One morning over a year past diagnosis, I was in New York City for a conference and had plans to meet my then-editor from the *New York Times* for breakfast. I was staying in midtown and our chosen breakfast spot was in the Village—not a complicated trip, if you know New York. But my visit coincided with intermittent subway breakdowns and I didn't want to get indefinitely stuck in a tunnel, so I ruled out the subway. Cabs weren't coming by the hotel to get fares, and I tried a rideshare, but the driver went to the wrong location. I should have hopped on the subway, but I couldn't make a decision. I had to call Arthur to help me think through this very simple problem.

As he and I talked, a cab pulled up in front of the hotel, and I got in. In the end, my transportation dilemma worked itself out, or so it seemed.

The thing is, the day before I had been an invited speaker at a conference on digital medicine. I had talked energetically with vendors and schmoozed during the cocktail hour, but the morning after, I couldn't think my way through taking the subway a few stops. I got to breakfast late. My editor was gracious, but the feeling of upset lingered. Cancer had, of all possible side effects, thoroughly discombobulated me.

I could sometimes feel the exhaustion like a harpy perched on my right shoulder, waiting. Waiting for what, I never knew. If I exercised, I would feel alert and happy for the rest of the day, but the next morning I might struggle to wake up, get out of bed, write, work. Then again, I might feel fine. At times, cooking restored my energy, but at other times the recipe I was using might as well have been written in code. I would give up and Arthur would take over.

I want to be wholly healed after my cancer treatment, and I'm not. As trade-offs go, there are a lot worse examples than fatigue, I know, just in health care: organ transplant patients who have to take immune suppressing medications for the rest of their lives, amputees whose natural limbs are replaced with prostheses, and kidney failure patients who would die without regular dialysis. Illness cannot always be fixed, which is another reason why we need care to be compassionate.

So, I am grateful that treatment saved my life. I am. Sometimes I'm also frustrated at what it took away.

TWENTY-EIGHT

Figures of Speech

THE UNIVERSITY OF Pittsburgh School of Public Health selected *The Emperor of All Maladies: A Biography of Cancer* as the book the entire school would read and discuss during the academic year that I was diagnosed with breast cancer. I had been invited to give a talk about the book and had accepted the invitation before I was diagnosed. Do you know the book? It won a Pulitzer, became a PBS *Frontline* series, and chronicles the efforts of heroic cancer researchers over the past several decades, as well as the lives of some patients. The author is Siddhartha Mukherjee, an oncologist. I read it soon after it came out and liked it.

I decided to go forward with the talk despite having become a cancer patient only months before. The evening arrived and I took the lecturer's spot in a classroom where the seats sloped steeply up so that, standing at the bottom, I felt small and vulnerable. People came in and were friendly, some even enthusiastic. I planned to talk about pink and believe it or not,

I wore pink, but not princess pink. I wore a skirt suit made of a deep purple fabric imprinted with neon-pink polka dots. Pink as rebellion, as showing off.

I talked about how we dress up cancer in metaphors—an idea that Susan Sontag first posited in her book *Illness as Metaphor* after being diagnosed with breast cancer. One metaphor that Sontag focuses on, and that often came up when I worked as an oncology nurse, is equating cancer treatment with being in a battle. No other common disease that I can think of is described this way: not heart disease, COPD, MS, Alzheimer's, ALS. Those are just diseases. The war metaphor makes cancer scarier than it might be otherwise, Sontag writes in *Illness as Metaphor*: "The effect of the military imagery on thinking about sickness and health is far from inconsequential. It overmobilizes, it overdescribes . . .We are not being invaded. The body is not a battlefield. The ill are neither unavoidable casualties nor the enemy. We—medicine, society—are not authorized to fight back by any means whatever." The word *invaded* interests me here since my cancer is medically labeled "invasive." Before I knew what that meant in the context of breast cancer—that the cancer had spread from the milk duct to surrounding breast tissue—it scared me. It sounded like I was "being invaded," but was I? Invasions come from outside known borders: armies invade countries, some viruses invade respiratory passages. My cancer arose from my tissue, my genes; in some sense my cancer *is* me. So, while cancer can be invasive, it is not an invasion but a failure of genes to brake when they should have. Limiting cancer's invasiveness and metastatic spread is not the same as fighting a war, and yet battle imagery for cancer persists.

Being afraid of cancer is normal. However, a school of thought asserts that cancer can be controlled by the power of positive thinking, as if patients' attitudes are a form of treatment in and of themselves. Sontag talked about this, and Barbara Ehrenreich updates Sontag's analysis in *Bright-Sided: How Positive Thinking Is Undermining America*. Ehrenreich says the idea that positiveness can help conquer illness, and especially cancer, persists even in the medical community. She encountered this attitude during treatment for her own breast cancer: "There was, I learned, an urgent medical reason to embrace cancer with a smile: a 'positive attitude' is supposedly essential to recovery." But the American Cancer Society says that feeling less than positive about one's life, and one's cancer, does not worsen the impact of the disease. It is true that chronic stress can depress the immune system, but that doesn't mean that happiness keeps people healthy; it means that in general, normal immune function is better maintained by people who live easier, more secure lives.

Because not everyone has a secure life, and thus the ability to be consistently happy, we can actually consider happiness to be a health disparity, what the Kaiser Family Foundation (KFF) defines as "differences in health and health care between groups that are closely linked with social, economic, and/ or environmental disadvantage." Data now shows that relative wealth and racial background mostly account for the real divides between patients who recover well from illnesses and those who don't: "Infant mortality rates are higher for Blacks and American Indians and Alaska Natives compared to whites, and Black males have the shortest life expectancy compared to other groups. Low-income people of all races report worse health status than higher income individuals." Attitude matters so much less to people's health than socioeconomic status, race, and ethnicity.

Back to *The Emperor of All Maladies*. During my talk, I analyzed the book through the lens of "The Emperor's New Clothes." You know the story. Two tailors who are con artists convince an emperor that not only do they sew the world's most beautiful clothes, but that the ability to see the clothes depends on viewers' refinement and intelligence. The uncouth and dim will not see the clothes at all, the tailors say.

The tailors cut the (nonexistent) cloth for the emperor's new clothes, fit the nonexistent garments to the emperor just so, and then parade the emperor among his subjects in his underwear. None of the emperor's advisers or any member of the populace speaks up for fear of being revealed as ignorant. Finally, a small child states the obvious: "He doesn't have anything on."

I brought this fairy tale up in my talk at the School of Public Health because calling cancer the "Emperor of all Maladies" introduces another metaphor. I had been diagnosed with the "emperor of all maladies." As an oncology nurse I was fine with that label for cancer, but Theresa the patient disliked it. Taking a book's title personally is probably a mistake, but the metaphor "emperor of all maladies" elevates cancer to preeminence among all illnesses, and that frightened me after my diagnosis. No one wants their stroke described as the Sovereign of All Sicknesses, their life-threatening heart attack the Autocrat of All Ailments. In my talk at the School of Public Health I argued that if we stripped cancer of its encumbering metaphors, it would be less scary, less oppressive. I also said that the *Emperor of All Maladies* is not dissimilar to "The Emperor's New Clothes," the idea being that it takes the guilelessness of a child to point out that underneath all the metaphors for cancer we have a centuries-old disease, naked and exposed. I argued that "Naked Cancer" would have less power over patients' minds than cancer distorted by metaphors. If we could see the cancer metaphors for the empty words they are and admit that without being called stupid (unlike the emperor's subjects in "The Emperor's New Clothes"), having cancer would be a slightly better experience. That sounds good and I even briefly owned the web domain Naked Cancer, not because I had hit on a great idea, but because I wanted *my* cancer to be less scary *to me*. I wanted to expose cancer as puny and ridiculous to make myself feel better, except that cancer is not a foolish emperor in a children's story promenading in his underwear, but a real and serious disease. Cancer exposed is still cancer.

Looking straight on at cancer unencumbered by metaphors of war or positive thinking or illness supremacy could have one important benefit: it might allow cancer patients to communicate more freely about their disease. The American Cancer Society recommends the sharing of feelings as a way to reduce the emotional burden of cancer: "A person with cancer should talk about their feelings . . . Working through their feelings can help a person with cancer feel more optimistic. And this optimism can lead to a better quality of life." Optimism sounds a bit like "Being Positive," but I don't think it's meant that way. The American Cancer Society website implicitly contrasts "optimism" with "sadness, distress, depression, fear, and anxiety." Optimism for cancer patients is the opposite of hopelessness.

And speaking of hopelessness, here's another figure of speech sometimes used in health care: "Slip through the cracks." I was working in home hospice one December, before my own diagnosis, and went to see a patient with chronic obstructive pulmonary disease, or COPD. He needed oxygen to be comfortable—without it he felt short of breath. The hospice had promised to deliver a new home oxygen machine to him since the one he had wasn't working well, but the new machine failed to arrive. The patient's wife, who had put up Christmas decorations on every bit of empty wall in their small house, was told, when she asked about the new oxygen concentrator that never got dropped off, "Sometimes people slip through the cracks."

The wife was furious and I agreed with her—not only about not getting the oxygen concentrator, but also about being so cavalierly brushed off. I did not want to believe that someone in the company I worked for had said such a thing, but I knew this couple to be honest, and why would they make the story up? I made sure the new concentrator would be delivered that day, as soon as possible, and was relieved to learn that the patient had done OK with the old one. I apologized, of course, and agreed to move the wife's complaint up the management chain.

There's another odd wrinkle here. Pittsburgh can be confusing; house numbers can be out of order numerically and some alleys have street names that are part of individual personal addresses. This couple's house opened off a wide alley, and had the *exact same house number* as the house next to theirs, that fronted on the street the alley came off. No one had noted this peculiarity anywhere in the chart. Was the oxygen concentrator delivered to the wrong house? I don't know—my manager would figure it out—but I wrote an email detailing what happened with the oxygen concentrator and explained the address issue. I also made an emotional plea, asking everyone to please, never ever tell a patient or family member that they "slipped through the cracks." Surely we could do better than that.

Not only can health care do better, it should, if clinicians want to give patients the best possible care. "[Compassionomics] is the scientific evidence that caring makes a difference," write Stephen Trzeciak and Anthony Mazzarelli in the introduction to their book *Compassionomics*. The claim that compassion's benefits can be objectively, or scientifically, validated makes their argument important for everyone involved in health care, including upper levels of management. They say that care providers have no idea how powerful compassion can be and call it a "game-changer" for health care with solid intellectual bona fides: "The aim of this book is not to change people's hearts, but rather to change people's *minds*—by sharing the overwhelming scientific evidence about the effects of compassion on patient outcomes, patient safety, provider well-being, employee engagement, and organizational performance."

Later in the book they specifically discuss how compassionate care affects breast cancer patients, citing a study done at Johns Hopkins in 1999. The study had a very simple design: 210 women who were breast cancer survivors were divided into two groups. All the women would receive a scripted presentation of methods for treating metastatic disease, but the women in the second group would receive compassionate interventions at the beginning and end of the presentation. Breast cancer patients tend to score high on assessments of anxiety, but the anxiety scores of the women who were treated with deliberate compassion were lower than those of women in the control group.

Consider a different example, in an entirely different situation. A 2020 study by Kevin Binning in the journal *Psychological Science* showed that a simple intervention in first-year physics and biology classes produced effects that continued throughout students' entire four years of college. The intervention is called "ecological-belonging." Intended to combat self-defeating stereotypes, it involves telling students at the start of their college careers that it is normal to find college challenging and that most students adapt to the challenges and succeed. A responsive writing assignment was required and the students read stories that reinforced the theme of rising above adversity. The intervention was so effective that after four semesters the researchers decried the control group as unethical and dispensed with it: "The intervention was especially impactful among historically underperforming students, as it improved course grades for ethnic minorities in introductory biology and for women in introductory physics. Regardless of demographics, attendance in the intervention classroom predicted higher cumulative grade point averages two to four years later." A small miracle, or maybe even a big one.

Compassionomics suggests that compassion can produce similarly miraculous effects for patients and that the absence of compassion can be powerfully deleterious. Takotsubo cardiomyopathy is known more colloquially as "broken heart syndrome." It is a rare cardiac event, first diagnosed in Japan in 1990, in which the left ventricle of the heart, the body's primary pump, responds to an emotional or physical shock by ballooning out at its tip, taking on the shape of a tako-tsubo, a Japanese fishing pot. When the ventricle is in this shape it cannot effectively pump blood, and patients experience chest pain and shortness of breath and sometimes collapse. The condition is not fully understood, but is speculated to result from a surge in stress hormones. Patients are hospitalized and most recover fully, but it can take up to four weeks for normal heart function to return. Stress can literally break the human heart, although not irreparably if patients receive proper care.

It's not cancer that ought to be exposed, then, but our inability to show patients compassion. Simple phrases, and not ones about fighting wars or pasting smiles on patients' faces, will do as a start: "I know this is hard." "We are in this together." "I am here for you. I care."

PART FOUR

The Long Haul

TWENTY-NINE

Pronouncement

TO PRONOUNCE CORRECTLY means to say something the way it is supposed to be said. "Po-ta-to" has a long $\bar{a}$ sound in the middle, not a short a. The final s is silent for both words in "Des Moines." To pronounce can also mean to declare solemnly. The pronouncement might be important: Astronauts landed on the moon. Or it might be a pompous opinion: The food snob pronounced fast food inedible.

A pronouncement can also be a declaration of death. Hospice nurses are empowered to pronounce when a patient enrolled in hospice dies and that includes hospice patients who pass away at home or in nursing homes. The nurse makes sure the patient is actually dead by checking for a pulse, listening for breath sounds, and with a stethoscope hearing the absence of a heartbeat. No earthly silence resembles a dead body's internal quiet. After verifying the patient's death, the nurse calls the medical examiner or coroner, who "releases" the body to her or him. The nurse next calls the funeral home to arrange a pickup, if the family wants that. Hospice nurses have to satisfy county and state requirements governing the official record of a patient's decease. Most pronouncements also require the emotional work of comforting family and friends.

The first day of my first home hospice job, I got called at home at seven a.m. A family needed a nurse to pronounce. I had never done one on my own before, so the night-shift manager reviewed the steps with me over the phone. A pronouncement, unlike so much of health care, requires very little paperwork. There's nothing to charge for once the patient is dead.

I had taken a position as a weekend float nurse, so I could be, and was, sent anywhere in Pittsburgh or its suburbs. The pronouncement was needed in an outlying town, about thirty minutes from my house. How does one meet strangers in this situation? Like this: "Hi. I'm Theresa, the hospice nurse."

"He's in here," someone said, pointing towards a small room to the right of the main entryway. In another era it would have been called a parlor. I remembered to say, "I'm so sorry," before I went to see the patient. That seems obvious, but I worried about forgetting. The family was American, but the patient— the deceased—and his wife were Italian. I don't know if they had been in the U.S. for days, months, or years, but she spoke thickly accented English. He was thin and wasted by his illness, lying on a hospital bed piled up with blankets in a corner of the room.

The patient was dead, but I did what was required to make sure, using my stethoscope to listen to the unbeating heart, checking for an absent pulse, and doing both for at least a minute. Then I called the medical examiner. This was my first time calling the ME, but over time I learned that every call was the same. He (it was always a he) answered the phone and spoke so quickly I could not understand—at least this first time—at all.

"I'm sorry, what?"

And again, too fast. "I'm sorry, what?"

And again, until he slowed down enough that I could understand: "Any signs of foul play?"

I felt tempted to say, "You mean, like the axe in his head?" because the question seemed absurd, but I just said, "No." Then I gave the patient's date of birth, diagnosis, address, funeral home, and physician. The ME, or whoever in that office took these calls, released the body to me and I took down the ME's name for our paperwork. I called the funeral home, and they said they would send someone right away. Then I went into the kitchen to see the family.

They had the lights on over their kitchen island, but the rest of the area, including a sunken family room with a widescreen TV, was in shadow. Huddled in the half-dark, they struck me as a nice family. I felt a warmth from them and for them, these strangers. We talked about the patient, what his death meant to his wife. One younger child was present, a granddaughter. She looked at me and at her grandmother, the patient's wife, and said how bad she felt that she hadn't gone in to physically see her grandfather over the past couple of days when he was actively dying. She looked maybe eight years old, and dark curls framed her face, just like her grandmother's.

I looked at her and smiled. "Life's about the long haul, kiddo, not the final mile."

The wife wanted to sit in the room with her dead husband, just sit, alone, until the funeral home came to take him away, and because of that the family asked me to skip the regular postmortem care, which in his case would have meant a bath and probably changing his clothes.

One of the daughters stood apart from the others in the dark end of the kitchen, making quiet phone calls. The daughter-in-law invited me to stay and eat with them, at least have a coffee. Bite-sized rolls of pastry filled with poppyseeds had appeared on the island. To stay or go? My sense of professional obligation prodded me to leave. I already had another patient to see and I had a twelve-hour shift ahead of me. Of course, staying could have been my professional obligation, too, but it felt less pressing.

As I internally debated, staff from the funeral home arrived. I decided to leave. I hugged everyone, then put on my jacket over my dark blue scrubs and hung my bag on my shoulder. I shut the door of the house behind me, unlocked my car and got in, then pulled up my work email on my phone to learn where I would go next. I thought of the patient's wife—her short, wavy black hair with strands of gray, her sad dark eyes. I turned on the car and drove away as the funeral home workers readied the patient's body for their van.

To pronounce: to officially declare that someone is dead; to mark the end of a life.

It is the most and the least we do.

THIRTY

Survivor

STAY ALIVE WAS a popular board game I played as a child, a much simpler game than Immortals, the one the kids bought for Christmas the year of my diagnosis. In the old TV commercial for the game, four children on a beach see it wash up with the tide and decide to play. The gameboard is a square plastic platform that consists of orderly rows with holes. Strips of flat plastic that crisscross under the gameboard have irregularly spaced holes and tabs on both ends that stick out from the four sides of the board. Those tabs move the plastic strips back and forth as players push and pull them, opening up and closing off holes. To start, players place their colored marbles randomly across the board and, on every turn, pull or push one of the levers, hoping to sink other players' marbles and leave their own. The player with only her own marbles left on the gameboard wins. In the commercial, a kid, wearing a bucket hat, is the one with a marble still on top. He says, his voice inflected with surprise and awe, "I'm the sole survivor."

Now we have *Survivor*, the TV-show franchise that pits very fit strangers against one another on a beautiful and understood to be deserted island. One by one, or so I hear, contestants get voted off the island. I've never seen the show, but I wonder if at the end the one person remaining says, voice tinged with surprise and awe, "I'm the sole survivor."

We also have survivalists, people with bunkers in their backyards or basements stocked with a year's supply of canned goods, filtered water, guns and ammo. Preppers. These people are convinced the apocalypse is coming and they will be prepared. They're an inversion of the people in *Survivor*, since they already know they will be among the sole survivors. Instead of surprise and awe, they speak with righteous certitude.

Survival as game, survival as entertainment, survival as life-preserving hobby. None of these captures the ambiguity, and confusion, that for me cannot be separated from the phrase "I'm a cancer survivor," even though, apparently, I am. Cancer creates difficult circumlocutions. I *had* cancer, which makes me a "former" cancer patient, but I'm taking Tamoxifen and "it"—the cancer—could "come back," which leaves me unsure where I fall on the survivor scale. Instead of calling myself a cancer survivor, I say, "I'm OK now," with a smile and a nod of my head. I'm like a magician. "Nothing to see here," I say as I pull up my sleeves, careful not to show my surgical scar. I smile, to soothe other people's discomfort. I don't want anyone to feel sorry for me because if they seem worried on my behalf, I start to worry, too. "Had" and "have," "recurrence" and "cure," "life" and "death," start to feel slippery, like consequences separated from time. "I had cancer" feels nothing like "I have cancer."

I would never contradict someone who calls herself a cancer survivor; I just don't feel the label applies to me. Or maybe it doesn't apply to me *yet*. I can't quit the yearly mammograms, regular follow-up appointments, and daily Tamoxifen. I mean, I could, but I won't, so I also can't quit the worry, which sidles into my mind at strange times. The worst is when ads for drugs to treat metastatic breast cancer randomly pop up on the internet. I tell myself they're not targeted to me, but they might be, some day.

Statistics tell us that one in eight American women will be diagnosed with breast cancer over the course of a lifetime. A TV show called *Cancer Survivor* would start with eight women, and seven of them would leave the island. The one remaining would have felt a lump, been called back for a follow-up mammogram, had the biopsy that came back positive for malignancy. She would have surgery, get chemotherapy (maybe), and radiation if her surgery was a lumpectomy and not a mastectomy. No one wants to be the "sole survivor" on that island.

If it feels like I'm still surviving, can I call myself a survivor? That's the crux of the matter, the paradox. I'm still surviving. Present tense. I'm a cancer patient and will be for ten years, because I take Tamoxifen for five years, and then I'll take a different drug, called an aromatase inhibitor, for another five years. Aromatase is an enzyme central to the production of estrogen and aromatase inhibitors work well to prevent breast cancer recurrences in postmenopausal women. Maybe after those ten years, if I'm cancer-free, maybe then I will call myself a "survivor." I'm supposed to be cured, I think, since that's what makes me a "survivor." Except no one says "cured." They don't even talk about it: treatment gets outlined, its specific steps explained, but no one talks about an absolute end-point to having the disease.

Cancer patients are generally denied the decisiveness of "cure." Instead, we have more technical labels with more-or-less precise meanings:

Complete Response
Remission
Disease-free survival (DFS)
Relapse-free survival (RFS)
Stable-Disease

I know this because I never said "cure" to my patients on the bone-marrow transplant floor and I embraced the ethical correctness of withholding that powerful word. It was not possible to say that a leukemia patient was cured when he left the hospital, free of disease, after two months of treatment. Having no disease was good, but cured? One hundred percent cured? As in, like measles or mumps, that person could never get cancer again? No. Doesn't happen. No guarantees, no promises. That is why, sometimes, I suddenly feel the fear. That is also why, sometimes, I imagine that I never had breast cancer. *Did I really have breast cancer? Did I? Really?* I can't always face it. It seems so unlikely, and yet, I did.

THIRTY-ONE

A Body in Motion

I HAVEN'T YET mentioned Marin Sewel. Marin is technically not my friend—she's my personal trainer. Our relationship is based on my paying her to keep me in shape, or at least to keep me from getting physically old before my time. I grew up with the idea that money and human relationships should be kept separate because money contaminates relationships, always. That can be true, but regardless, Marin is my friend. I know and care about her life, and I'm pretty sure she feels the same.

Marin belongs in this book because she never wavered in her commitment to my working out. She never assumed I would be too tired or too sad to exercise. She never encouraged me to "take a break." It would have been so easy, but doing that, for me, would have felt like dereliction of personal duty. I took off the two weeks required after surgery and then was back in the gym, following the rules they gave me about not lifting too much, but doing whatever else I could. During radiation treatments, I would go to my workout, drive home, change into biking clothes, and ride to the hospital.

At a workout I told Marin I likely had breast cancer, and also at a workout I told her I definitely had cancer. I said that I wanted to keep coming to the gym. In some ways, it felt like the most important thing I would do following my diagnosis. I only have one body and it's the only body I will ever have. I could have said, *I hate you, body*—you let me down. Like that woman's T-shirt that said, printed across the chest: "Of course these are fake. My real ones tried to kill me." But turning my back on my body wouldn't make anything about my situation better. So, not *screw you, body*, but *screw you, cancer*. Cancer got part of my right breast, but I own my body.

My daughters are athletes, but I never was, having been raised at a time, in southwest Missouri, when girls could be smart or athletic, but not both. A stigma was attached to being a smart girl and a different stigma was attached to being athletic. I made my choice—the smart girl—but I am glad that my daughters have never had to settle in that way.

In my twenties, I discovered my own athleticism through college intramural sports, bike trips with Arthur, and lap swimming with friends and then on my own. I've also always been a big walker, and during the year I lived in Manhattan, when I got my master's degree in English at Columbia, I often took long walks in Riverside Park, watching colorfully dressed children playing soccer and couples lounging on blankets and, once, a nun jogging in a habit and tennis shoes.

Late in my forties my knees started to hurt doing what in health care we call activities of daily living. My kneecaps are off-center—apparently some people are born that way—which puts me at risk for injury and, I discovered, pain. The pain sent me to a trainer, who also became a friend. When he got married and moved away, I started working with Marin. It took time and careful work, but I can now do lunges and squats, sinking deep, and nothing hurts. I wasn't going to give that up because of cancer.

Marin got me to lift weights, do pushups, swing kettle-bells, breathe. She noted when my post-op strength returned to where it had been, and when I surpassed it *even though I had cancer*. After my diagnosis I strived to ensure that cancer would not sabotage my sense of who I physically was, and I may have cared about that more than the average person due to the effects of being on bedrest at the end of my twins' pregnancy. A standard uterus is designed to hold one baby, not two or more. At thirty-two weeks, the midwife told me I was beginning to dilate and needed to stay in bed. This was basic physics: bedrest would keep the weight of the two babies (plus amniotic fluid and the placenta) off the cervix, reducing the degree to which gravity affected the pregnancy.

Even before I was put on bedrest, though, I was told to "rest as much as possible." I had Conrad to care for, but beyond that, something as nonstrenuous as going for a walk was not allowed. The result of all this rest was two healthy babies born at thirty-four weeks, and a mom so weak I could barely walk one block. Muscle atrophy, or weakening from disuse, can begin within three days of a patient being immobilized, and in intensive care units, as many as 90 percent of patients will develop muscle atrophy during a lengthy hospitalization.

This phenomenon is often crudely summarized as "Use it or lose it."

It was all worth it, of course, because I ended up with two wonderful daughters. But once they were born, I was weak and felt broken, and I was breastfeeding two babies, caring for a toddler, and sleeping for five hours a night divided into chunks of two hours and three hours, if I was lucky. It is possible that I never again wanted to feel that overloaded while feeling physically capable of so little. I wouldn't rule it out. Or maybe I just didn't want my health problem to take over my whole life and my whole body. I didn't have a lot of choice when I was pregnant with Miranda and Sophia, but with breast cancer, I did.

Marin says the gym is one place where failure is good. If I lift a weight to the point where I cannot lift it one more time no matter how hard I try, that means I have fully taxed the muscle and it will be stronger afterwards as a result. I used to hate that feeling of having maxed out my strength, of trying to curl a dumbbell up to my shoulder one more time and not being able to. In time, though, I grew to like my lapses because they showed me where my edge was. Learning how much I could not lift set a challenge for the next time.

And maybe that's part of what I like, too—there's always a next time. A body in motion will stay in motion unless acted on by an outside force. That's Isaac Newton's first law of motion and foundational to the development of modern physics, although it was first formulated in 1686. Stay in motion. Use or lose it. Research shows that strength training keeps people feeling young. How counterproductive it would be to give that up because of cancer.

THIRTY-TWO

Just a Few Breast Cancer Patients Sitting Around Talking

MY FRIEND AND neighbor, U, asked several of her friends who had breast cancer to come together and share experiences. It's a little weird, the number of women she knows who have been diagnosed with this disease. She taught at a small high school and two other teachers in her department got breast cancer within a few years of U's diagnosis. Also, two of our near neighbors were recently diagnosed, which adds up to four women who live within one block of one another, all getting breast cancer at roughly the same time. Another woman was a colleague of U's husband. And I have a friend—who was not in our group, but still—younger than I am with a worse diagnosis, who learned of her disease maybe a year before I learned of mine. Why do so many women have breast cancer?

That was U's concern: why is breast cancer ubiquitous? Instead of money being spent on pink ribbons and encouraging women to get mammograms, she would like research done on whether pesticides and plastics are making the incidence of breast cancer rise in the developed world. Another member of the group, O, came through treatment OK, but developed a horrible rash and itching in response to one of the medications she was given, maybe. No one seems able to figure the rash out or control it, and she is suffering, but she thinks very little about her cancer because the rash and itching have driven it out of her mind. I am not sure she finds that a good bargain, similar to the patients who are cancer-free but can barely walk due to nerve damage from chemotherapy.

L responded to breast cancer with the same matter-of-factness she says she brings to every challenge in her life: if I need to worry about this, I will, but until then, I'm not worrying. Due to a death in the family A couldn't make our last meeting, but at the meeting before that, she spoke about her newfound ability to say no to things following her diagnosis of breast cancer. She had been given extra responsibility that she didn't like at her job, and after her diagnosis she told them she could no longer do the extra work. That inspired me like nothing else I heard from anyone in or outside the group. Cancer makes it possible to say no to things without feeling guilty—something nurses and women have a hard time doing. Finally, two of the group members dropped out because they didn't feel the need to talk about breast cancer with similarly diagnosed friends— fair enough.

And then there's me. When I first came to the group, I wanted to know how everyone had fared within the health care system, because I had painfully discovered that, despite the best efforts of good nurses and doctors, people did fall through the cracks all the time. Everyone's experiences were similar to mine; none of us received egregiously bad care, but we all felt that no health care professionals were really looking out for us. Contrast that with my much younger friend, who does not live in Pittsburgh, who felt very cared for, both immediately after her diagnosis and as she progressed through treatment. Her follow-up scan, biopsy, and start of treatment were all scheduled for her and occurred one right after the other. She did not have to stand in a hallway and lose her temper over the timing of her pathology results, only to be told by the nurse, "Well, I leave at four." And in general, she seemed calmer about treatment than any of the women in our breast cancer group, giving credence to arguments about the clinical advantages of compassion. A small amount of caring can have an outsize beneficial effect on how patients feel about themselves, their illness, and treatment.

Another thing about me is, I wrote this book. I have realized that writing a book about having cancer is not conducive to "putting cancer behind me." For that reason, I particularly enjoyed hearing that L doesn't think much about her diagnosis. U also has moved cancer from the front to the back of her mind, but for a completely different reason from L. U couldn't tolerate Tamoxifen or aromatase inhibitors—the drugs given to prevent breast cancer recurrences in postmenopausal women—because both classes of drugs gave her significant brain fog and made her short of breath (a rare side effect). She stopped taking the drugs and the side effects resolved almost immediately, but she's concerned about being off the medication. Of course, a friend of hers told U a story about another friend who didn't take Tamoxifen and had her breast cancer return.

Of course. I told U that people remember those stories because they stick out—we don't hear about the women who stop taking Tamoxifen and do OK, even though statistically they must exist in much larger numbers than the women whose breast cancer comes back.

Do you know the play *A Coupla White Chicks Sitting Around Talking*? It was written by John Ford Noonan and premiered in 1979 at the Astor Place Theater in New York, where it ran for more than eight hundred performances. It reads as a strange play, but I bet that onstage with the right actresses it's a knockout comedy. The only two characters are Maude Mix, an uptight Westchester County housewife, and Hannah Mae Bindler, Maude's new neighbor from Texas. Hannah Mae cajoles her way into Maude's life by showing up in Maude's kitchen around eleven a.m., insisting on coffee and conversation. The possible friendship between the two women leads Hannah Mae's husband, Carl Joe, to seduce Maude (offstage), hoping that jealousy will turn the women against one another. In this, Carl Joe has badly misjudged his wife: "The dumb cluck thinks he can come in here and . . . turn me back into his little Texas cheerleader. Well, look at us. Are we screaming at each other? Am I threatening to tear out your eyes? No."

The play keeps getting odder, but also more meaningful, as the relationship between the two women deepens over the course of a few days. In the final scene, they return to Maude's kitchen following a wild weekend spent together in New York City. The stage notes describe Maude as "completely transformed: hair restyled, spiked heels, tight suggestive dress, lots of jewelry, lipstick." Maude even tries to demolish her perfect

Better Homes and Gardens kitchen until Hannah Mae convinces her not to.

Nothing about this play resembles my cancer discussion group. Except: Creating friendship out of nothing more than a yearning to associate as women with a shared experience. Hannah Mae, new to Westchester County, wants a friend. Our group formed in response to our multiple breast cancer diagnoses, but we chose to talk to one another, connecting over U's home-baked treats and hot tea, similar to how Maude and Hannah Mae connect over cake and coffee. I'm not sure why Noonan described Maude and Hannah Mae as "white chicks." What that phrase meant in 1979 differs from how it might come across now, but the women superficially fall into easy stereotypes: Maude is a white, upper-middle-class, slightly robotic East Coast homemaker, and Hannah Mae is a Southern Belle, with a Texas twist that means she won't take no for an answer. I suppose it is the idea that, as one review said, opposites attract, and Maude and Hannah Mae are very different from each other.

Something about the play pulls at me, despite its dated-feeling call-out to "white chicks." Maude decided that she and Hannah Mae had to go to New York City for the weekend because Maude's husband dumped her for a younger woman. That is not the same as having cancer, but cancer, and breast cancer especially for women, feels like a betrayal. Our cells broke the rules, let us down, put our lives at risk, and we could not say about them, as Hannah Mae did Carl Joe, "Those dumb clucks." I can imagine myself as Maude, distraught, going off to Manhattan with a friend and returning with a cutting-edge hairstyle and wearing stiletto heels, as if becoming a new version of myself would save me from cancer.

Maybe that's what friends do when we're diagnosed: keep us company, hold us steady. I remember when U told me she had breast cancer. I went to her house as soon as I could and we sat in her backyard, under her apple tree, on a sunny June day, and talked over everything she had been told and how she felt. Her friends, who were diagnosed before she was, told her what to expect from treatment. L, who got breast cancer after the rest of us, gathered advice from the group on different medical oncologists and where to have her radiation treatments. We didn't meet that often, only a few times in total, and some of us, who are writers of one kind or another, did a reading together. However, the group calmed me. It showed me that I would get through treatment, and that there were as many ways of doing that as there were women being diagnosed with breast cancer.

THIRTY-THREE

Back to Work

AFTER I'D BEEN on Tamoxifen for three months and a bit, and I felt less tired and mentally sharper, I got my old job back, working as a fill-in home hospice nurse two days every week. I hadn't been gone that long, but it seemed like everything had changed. The corporate headquarters—where I would go for my reorientation—was now located in a far Pittsburgh suburb, in a bland two-story office building in the middle of a parking lot. It was set back from the road, like the surrounding bland office buildings with wide driveways curving through carefully mowed lawns. The rent must have been cheap. Why else would anyone have an office in the middle of suburban nowhere?

The hospice company had the first floor of the building, part of which was built into a low hill that put some of the offices underground. New staff described as "schedulers" worked in the largest of the underground, and therefore window-less, rooms. They hunched in cubicles, staring into computer screens. I honestly do not know what they did at the company, but the arrangement seemed really depressing. A job is a job, I guess, but their, to me, grim workspace might have been a clue that the company had changed more than I realized. In the old space, in Pittsburgh proper, there had been windows. Of course people work in basements, but the lack of windows felt stark. Hospice workers need the light.

I came to learn that the alterations really began when a holding company bought the hospice a few months before I went on leave. Not much was different immediately with that switch, at least not that I noticed, but I deliberately tried to remain ignorant of the details of the buyout, a coping strategy I would not recommend. Because when I returned, it seemed that the hospice was not only a for-profit company on paper but an actual for-profit company. I may have been naïve—what company is ever only for-profit on paper?—but I had had a couple of phone calls with the former president and admired his commitment. He wanted us to be the best hospice ever. I doubt that anyone at the holding company ever gave a thought to that idea.

While I was on leave, the company closed their inpatient hospice facility. The closure got a write-up in the Pittsburgh paper and the official reason given for shutting the unit down was that beds were often unfilled, indicating that the facility was underused. The true reason, I found out later, was that the inpatient unit wasn't profitable *on its own*. Many of our hospice volunteers quit in response to the closure. They wanted to show their displeasure with nickel-and-diming of the dying. That's how it is, though, in the social Darwinist world of for-profit health care. Interventions are evaluated in terms of the amount of money they bring in.

Wait a minute, though. Let's back up. I had told myself I would never work as a nurse in a for-profit company. Never. But I knew one of the attending physicians at this new for-profit hospice and respected him tremendously. He became the chief medical officer and I thought he would be a bulwark against profiteering. I was wrong about that. He tried, but his trying didn't make a difference after the holding company bought the hospice—at least that's how the timeline looked to me. People who run companies to make money, who buy companies to, as they say, diversify their portfolios, may not care at all about the actual work those companies do. The higher-ups said they cared about quality and about patients, and maybe they did, but they seemed to care more about meeting their budgets, hitting their revenue goals, maximizing their monetary incentives, and keeping their labor costs—that primarily means nurses—low.

I returned, though, and at first I didn't pay attention to the overall penny-pinching feel of the place. I would have a week of reorientation and then be out in the field, learning from another nurse. At orientation I kept saying how glad I was to be back. It felt good, I think. But the windowless offices, the training room that was too small to hold all of the new hires in my group, the nurse educator who also worked full-time as a manager because the company had a hard time keeping staff, raised questions I guessed I would not like the answers to.

I wanted this chapter to be triumphant, a celebration of my return to nursing, despite Tamoxifen clouding my brain. With this company, though, and this job, I quickly saw that there was little to celebrate. The hard part, the sad part, is that so many jobs in health care are now like this. One small but telling example: the company changed the way they reimbursed for gas and as a result I no longer got compensated for the gas I used on the job and was never paid for mileage. They started sending me on wild goose chases, without explaining why. I would visit patient x at the hospital and try to start them on hospice. Then I had to see patient y, who just got admitted to the emergency department. I was being paid per visit, rather than by the hour, so these time-consuming visits probably saved the company money. I'm sure that each visit checked some bureaucratic box put in place by the Centers for Medicare & Medicaid Services and monitored by a staff member working in the windowless room. Much of the nurses' record-keeping focused on dotting our i's and crossing our t's so that payments would come in on time.

I met great nurses working for this company. Great nurses with too many patients and too much paperwork. Nurses who finished their electronic charting in the evenings at home every night they worked but weren't paid for that time because they were salaried employees. Nurses whose burden of required emails grew and grew, because the electronic record system was designed for the people in the windowless room, not those of us out in the field working with patients.

Americans used to have the best health care in the world and the myth persists that we still do, but compared to other industrialized countries, our health care is mediocre in many areas, even though we also spend more than those other countries to get worse care overall. Health care has become big business over the past several decades, creating large profits for insurance company CEOs, drug companies, device manufacturers, and executives of large hospital systems, while putting humane, respectful care on the back burner. But no one can serve two masters. It's worth revisiting the actual Biblical quotation, Matthew 6:24, because the full meaning matters: "No one can serve two masters; for either he will hate the one and love the other, or else he will be loyal to the one and despise the other. You cannot serve God and mammon." It's not clear that making money and treating patients with compassion are mutually exclusive, but our existing system seems to suppose they are. A modern revision of Matthew would read, "One cannot serve both patients and profits," and the sick deserve compassion, industry, and commitment, every single one.

Here is the story of one patient. I'll call him Dan. Dan loved motorcycles and Clint Eastwood movies. He named his cat Hog, after his Harley, and he joked that his cat was trying to kill him by kinking his oxygen tubing. Dan had congestive heart failure and more than once his wife bitterly told me the story of how, after his diagnosis, he put his supplemental oxygen aside and took his bike out one final time. His last ever ride on his Harley.

Dan was one of the few patients I'd cared for who was still on service when I returned from my leave. He said, "We haven't seen you for a while." And I thought about it, and then I told them—him and his wife. *Breast cancer.* Most people, patients, I wouldn't tell, but I decided that Dan deserved the true story.

It would not be lying to say that caregiving can feel like love even when the two people are strangers, even when, or maybe especially because, one of them is dying. That is the promise of hospice, or should be. And this is why for-profit hospices are just plain wrong, because money those companies could put into improving patient care goes to shareholders or owners, instead. Capitalism is supposed to encourage streamlining, but in this company, at least, it felt like siphoning. Not that Dan in particular was denied services or medications he needed, but my mandate seemed to be *hurry, hurry, hurry.* Finish the visit, chart on the computer, move on to the next patient so that I could see as many people as possible in one day.

I and the licensed practical nurse (LPN) on our team saw patients for the regular nurses, who maintained patient caseloads well above the usual home hospice standards. The point of home hospice care is for the patient and family to develop a trusting relationship with one nurse, not to have that nurse constantly replaced by someone who gets paid less. One case manager often worked on her day off to keep up with her large caseload. Some might call that dedication, but really, her generosity was being exploited. The company cared little about staff well-being, or making sure that every patient got the personal attention they needed.

A situational blindness to dysfunction develops in almost everyone who works in health care. It's what enables us to keep doing the work. Some people acclimate to it better than others and that is what I always tried to do. To not count the cost. Being on the other side due to cancer showed me that one person, working alone, trying as hard as she can, cannot make up for the lack of humanity in the system. I told myself that by giving 120 percent to all my patients I could balance out the

50 percent from the health care system, but a middle-schooler could see that the math doesn't work out.

That is especially true when the electronic system of charting we nurses used—how we recorded the facts of the visit on a tablet—required more concentrated time and attention than I was ever told to give patients. Here is what I had to do after leaving a patient's home, i.e. at the end of a visit. Actually, before I left, I would have the patient, or their caregiver, sign my electronic tablet to verify that I made the visit. The tablet would automatically record how long the visit was because I had electronically "initiated the visit" when I first got to the patient's house. Visits of too short a duration had to be justified on a separate menu with a reason, such as, "patient was going out to lunch" or "patient felt tired and wanted to take a nap." Afterwards, in my car, I was supposed to complete the paperwork on my tablet, and I would if I had time. I had to be quick, but also couldn't make a mistake filling out the multitude of required drop-down menus with tiny boxes because that could hold up a payment. When I finished the charting, I would also sign the computer, verifying, I guess, that I was actually me. Nothing was more important than paperwork done well.

It might not sound so bad, but I was taking care of people who were dying. If I still had tears, they would stain this page. All I wanted was to be a good nurse.

THIRTY-FOUR

Turtles

IN JUNE WE took a family bike trip, intending to ride the trail that goes all the way from Pittsburgh to Washington, DC, along repurposed towpaths and former railbeds. It's a long trip, but we knew people who had done it in five days and that seemed possible, especially since we cut off a bit at the start and planned to cut off a bit at the end, making it about three hundred miles in total. Conrad volunteered to drive along the route and carry our stuff. He was our SAG wagon: support and gear. It was a good way for someone who hates exercise to still be included.

I figured the trip would be hard for me, which was why I wanted a SAG wagon. There was a time when I could have hopped on my bike and ridden sixty miles of flat road, no problem, in a single day. That time was before Tamoxifen, and I worried I would have the same trouble on the bike that I had when we hiked at Harper's Ferry.

The first day, I stopped before the end of the ride and instead rode in the car with Conrad to where we had planned to stay that night. Doing fifty-five miles in one day under my own steam ended up being impossible. I had no reserves. The second day of riding, I grew frustrated at my own inability to brute-force my way through, when, as happened the day before, I hit thirty miles and could not go farther. Conrad again picked me up, along with Sophia, who had developed a cold and wasn't feeling great. Arthur and Miranda kept going on the path and all five of us met up a few hours later in Cumberland, Maryland.

The third day of the trip we woke up to rain in Cumberland and a forecast of rain for the entire day. It would be our first day on the Chesapeake & Ohio, or as everyone calls it, the C&O, the trail that goes from Cumberland to Washington, DC. We had heard it was a more difficult ride than the trail that ended in Cumberland, called the Great Allegheny Passage, or GAP trail. The C&O was less well cared for, narrower, rougher. So, we knew the new path would be challenging, but we hadn't understood about the rain. It had been raining off and on for days. It had rained and rained and rained, and it was still raining.

Conrad had returned to Pittsburgh for a friend's graduation party and Sophia, who'd started to feel worse, went with him to rest and get a good night's sleep. We were to meet up at the next stop, in Maryland, at the end of the day of riding.

That morning in Cumberland, Arthur, Miranda, and I set out. I've ridden in rain quite a bit, down the Oregon coast, flanked by logging trucks and RVs that lumbered up hills. Also, in Wisconsin and Michigan, when Arthur and I, leaving from Chicago, rode our bikes all the way around Lake Michigan. Also here in Pittsburgh, when I rode to and from nursing school, to and from the hospital, to and from radiation treatments. Rain can be tolerable if you've got rain gear and paved trails. The C&O trail, though, was packed gravel surrounded on both sides by a verge of waist-high grass, blooming honeysuckle, and cattails that rose up taller than my head. The gravel path was only wide enough for one bike at a time, and small puddles dotted it here and there. In many spots it was more dirt than gravel and the rain was transforming the dirt into mud.

When we first got on the path I saw a turtle bigger than my head sitting on a tree root. It looked like it was going places, but very slowly—kind of like us, in the mud and rain. As I splashed through puddle after puddle on the path, I told myself that that was how the day would go—it would be wet. It wasn't cold, and the scenery was lush: small purple-and-white flowers poked out of bright green grasses, and climbing vines swirled around high trees. The old canal, what had been the C&O, was on our left, filled with stagnant water carpeted with bright yellow pollen. The Potomac River flowed by on our right.

The rain kept falling and we kept going, sometimes encountering long trenches of mud hiding deep ruts left by riders before us. I noticed that the water in the old canal, on our left, was only about five inches below the level of the bike path. I looked at the trees in a new way—could we climb them if we needed shelter? There were no low branches, and the slender green vines encircling them would not have held our weight. I thought about how people in books and movies climb trees to save their lives. I wondered how easy it really is to climb a tree.

Riding just behind me, Miranda called, "Is anyone else concerned by this water on our left?"

"Yes," I said. Yelling back and forth, we talked about the trees, how we were unlikely to find safe purchase along their branchless trunks. We came to a puddle that extended thirty feet along the path and all three of us got stuck in the mud. There was nothing for it—we had to get off and walk. There was mud and rain and no shelter and the rain had turned heavy and cold. I worried we had crossed over the line between committed and foolish.

"They get flash floods along the bike path," a man in the hotel restaurant had told us that morning, with what looked like a gleeful grin, as if he wanted to scare us, or as if he thought us ridiculous for biking in the rain when sensible people would have stayed inside. Maybe he was trying to warn us but didn't get the tone right. He might not have known how to tell three strangers who were obviously from out of town: "Don't ride today—it's dangerous." We would sometimes hear machinery to our left, and we crossed the occasional lonely country road. Once there was even a house, except it looked like no one was home.

At the next break in the trail, there was a parking lot and a sodden open campground. We stopped and stood in the rain, deciding what to do. The Potomac roared by, close to level with the campground, but not the path. It was a sheet of gray, moving violently fast. Oldtown, the next town on the path, was six miles away. On a normal day that would be an easy thirty-minute ride. With the rain and mud, it would probably take an hour, but we would at least have shelter there. We didn't have our SAG wagon because Conrad had stayed in Pittsburgh overnight, but cell reception was so poor along the trail that we likely couldn't have reached him even if he had been in Cumberland.

It had taken us two hours to ride the ten miles from Cumberland to the campground. Going back seemed like a terrible idea considering how close the canal water had come to the trail in spots on our ride out. Two additional hours of rain might have completely flooded sections of the path. But we also thought, irrationally, that Oldtown didn't sound promising. We joked about calling a cab, a Lyft or an Uber.

Then a pickup truck pulled into the campground. The driver told us the trail on the way to Oldtown was flooded. His passengers, in the back seat of the four-door pickup, were two bike riders who said they had been rescued by the driver. That was the word they used: rescued. We asked about biking on the nearby highway to Oldtown, off the trail. They said branches had fallen on the road already and with the wind and rain it wasn't safe. The best thing, they said, would be for us to ride the ten miles back to Cumberland on the trail, a prospect that felt undoable.

They pulled out of the parking lot, leaving us uncertain and forlorn, but another pickup truck pulled in very soon after. We talked about asking him for a ride. I'm not good at that—asking for help. Being a nurse means I help other people. But he stopped, rolled down his window, and I asked. I said we could pay him, but he declined that offer right away. I said we would get his truck dirty and he said that dirt never hurt nothin', that it didn't matter at all. He helped us pile our three bikes in the back of the truck. Then we got into the backseat of the cab, dirty and wet, but luxuriously out of the rain.

The cab had the acrid scent of cigarette smoke, and it combined with our sweat and the earthy smell of mud. The driver told us that local people were driving back and forth on the highway, checking the trail, looking out for bicyclists. "You're a lifesaver," I told the driver and it felt true even if it wasn't literally true. Who knows, though, maybe it was. People hadn't had rain like that in a long time, the driver said—all the creeks and streams were overflowing. He dropped us off in Cumberland in the parking lot of the hotel we had left that morning. Arthur tried again to pay him, but he refused. "I was happy to do it and I'd do it again," he said. We didn't exchange names—an oversight I still regret.

By the next day a warning, in red on the National Park Service website, declared that multiple sections of the bike path were underwater and extreme caution was advised. The whole section of Maryland and Virginia that the bike path cut through was swollen with water: creeks rose, the Potomac burst its banks, and bridges and pathways got washed away. I found a picture online of Harper's Ferry, one of our upcoming stops, and the bike path was submerged beneath three feet of water.

There were no rooms in the hotel where we had spent the night before, so I called a different hotel in Cumberland and got a room. We rode by the local bike shop and used the outside hose there to blast caked-on sludge off our bikes and off ourselves. The new hotel was next to the bike shop and we walked our bikes over in the rain. The hotel lobby was bright and warm, decorated with large backlit photographs of flowers. It felt like the opposite of everything we had gone through on the trail. It was clean, dry, and safe. In the room I took off my bike gloves and realized I could barely feel my fingertips. When undressing for a hot shower, I saw that my white socks had turned black from the mud and I threw them away, as if they were contaminated. Then I stepped into the warm water and watched mud trail down my legs. It left a pattern of silt on the bathtub floor.

After Miranda and Arthur showered, we had lunch at the closest local place. I didn't feel hungry, but I ate just the same. *We* ate just the same. We all felt cold, like we just couldn't warm up, so back in the room we turned up the heat, slid between the clean, dry sheets, pulled blankets up to our chins, and slept. We slept through Conrad's text giving his estimated arrival time at the hotel and his texted updates. We slept until his knocking on the hotel room door woke us. Sophia had stayed in Pittsburgh after developing a fever. Our family bike trip to DC clearly was not meant to be.

DURING THE RIDE that last day, looking for shelter from the rain, we had stopped where an old canal house and lock still stand. There wasn't any shelter, but we met two men, and since I'm not great at directions, I prodded Arthur to ask them for advice. Should we stay on the bike path or try the road? We intended to reach a town roughly fifty miles away. Arthur found out that the men were turtle researchers. Imagine that. They told Arthur that an increase in biodiversity always followed flooding in the area, which was part of why the C&O path and its environs were a good habitat for turtles. Maryland, in fact, is home to nineteen different species of turtle, including snapping turtles and softshell turtles. The area where we were on the path is home to Eastern box turtles and painted turtles, but I don't know which turtles they were looking for.

Each of those turtles has an interesting feature. The box turtle's bottom shell functions like a drawbridge when a predator attacks. The turtle pulls its head and four legs into its upper shell and then draws up the lower shell till it connects with the lower edge of the upper shell, creating a seal all the way around the turtle that a predator cannot break. Painted turtles have their own biological trick. When they hibernate in winter, they can't take in enough oxygen to stay alive and out of necessity switch to anaerobic (without oxygen) respiration instead, producing lactic acid. Excess lactic acid is dangerous in turtles (and humans), but painted turtles neutralize the lactic acid made during hibernation with calcium and magnesium from their shells. Their shells keep them metabolically balanced while they wait out the most difficult weeks of winter.

In response to Arthur's request for their opinion, the older of the two researchers said we could take the road but it had blind twists and turns and no shoulder. He recommended continuing on the bike path, so we got back on our bikes and rode off, immediately passing a small turtle, the size of my fist, angled up on its side in the high grass. The Maryland turtles were not the helpless-seeming pet store turtles of my childhood—these turtles intended to survive.

We saw the turtle researchers two more times, once on the path, where I shouted, "It's us again—right behind you." They looked back at us, smiling, so happy to be walking in the rain, talking about turtles. The next time we saw them was when they were leaving the parking lot at Pigmans Ferry, where we ended our ride. The older researcher waved to us as he pulled out of the parking lot and said we would probably meet up again at the next stop on the trail. But our trip was over, even though we didn't know it yet. There were no signs that the rain would stop, and regardless, the water on the path would not clear for days. A week after our trip, large sections of the trail still remained closed.

After Conrad arrived at the hotel in Cumberland, the four of us went out to dinner. Then we put the bikes on the car rack, loaded up the rest of our gear, some of which was still soaking wet and covered in mud, and drove home. I felt impossibly tired. Our vacation had imploded. If only I could have ridden out the storm—or my cancer—by drawing into a shell or nestling in the mud while my body's chemical magic kept me safe.

THIRTY-FIVE

One-Year Mammogram

ACTIVE CANCER TREATMENT ends, but not surveillance. I had follow-up appointments, separated by a few months, with the medical oncologist and the radiation oncologist after my treatment finished. My MedOnc said the visits were to see how I was doing and to make sure I kept taking Tamoxifen, which made me feel a bit like a child. I would have told my doctors if I stopped taking Tam.

In addition to the regular doctor's visits, I would of course have a yearly mammogram. There's nothing like an annual scan *after* a cancer diagnosis: the opportunity to relive the trauma of going in for a medical test and leaving diagnosed with what can be a fatal disease. I even thought about getting my mammograms at a different hospital, one where I hadn't been diagnosed with breast cancer. I tried that, but the available times were less convenient so I returned to the hospital where I was diagnosed. I may try a new location another time, but I wonder if having my imaging done in an unfamiliar place would lessen my fear, or just make it different.

I scheduled my first-year mammogram for when I was supposed to—early fall. And doing that, only that, made me anxious. For some reason I agreed to a routine scan, rather than a "diagnostic mammogram." A routine mammogram requires another, later appointment if the radiologist sees anything concerning, whereas with a diagnostic screen, any additional imaging is done that day and read by the radiologist, who discusses the result with the patient before she leaves. From now on I plan to try to always have a diagnostic mammogram, and how that first mammogram went explains why.

I had the mammogram on the Wednesday before Labor Day weekend. I knew the imaging department wouldn't give results over the weekend or on Labor Day, so I expected the reading by Friday at the latest to avoid waiting three extra days for the results. I was also part of a study on combining mammography with ultrasound, which I supposed made a timely reading more likely. That is, I thought that my first mammogram after diagnosis would be flagged in some way to alert someone that in the interests of compassion I should get my result quickly, and I defined quickly as "in two days rather than six." *Why* I thought that puzzles me now, since my experience of DIY cancer care should have taught me otherwise, but I did believe that such kindness would be built into the system, probably because my "routine" mammogram was not ordinary to me.

Friday came and I sent an email to the research coordinator in the morning saying I very much hoped for the results of my mammogram that day.

In the final line of the email I wrote, "My worry about breast cancer does not take a holiday." This reads as overly dramatic to me, and the entire email was brusque in a way I normally wouldn't be, but I was anxious and knew that every day spent waiting for the result would increase my concern. If I had only considered statistics, I would not have worried, should not have, because the chances of my cancer recurring after one year were basically nil. But I was living in the realm of worst-case what-ifs: what if my cancer came back? What if I have a new cancer?

The research coordinator wrote back saying she understood and that two radiologists were reading my mammogram right then. As soon as she had "integrated" the results I would get the reading. Great. By the end of the day, I would know whether I was clear or if I needed to return for repeat imaging. But by 3:50 p.m. that same day I had not heard anything. I was very anxious, imagining really dumb things, such as, my result was so terrible they didn't know how to tell me. I wrote again with a nudge and at 4:51 p.m. I learned that "It's delayed" and "Nevertheless, it's not up to my control whether I get the radiologist's reading results on time ... unfortunately we're helpless to get the information received at our end." I wrote back and said her email was the lousiest nonapology I had ever heard. A few more emails, including from the MD running the study, went back and forth, spelling out problems with locked doors, absent employees, and difficult computers. The physician running the study complained about staff at the cancer center being unexpectedly away and "the computers are still not cooperating." In one message I told the research coordinator to "do your damn job," which led the physician to chide me for being abusive to her staff.

By the end of that evening, my fear of a recurrence, irrational or not, and my anger, justified or not, left me desperately anxious and unable to focus on anything else. It was Arthur, who never uses social media, who urged me to take my complaint to Twitter. I did. The next day, Saturday, the head of the radiology department called me on my cell phone. She apologized for the delay in getting me my result and said she had read the entire email chain between me and the study staff. Something in her voice told me that she agreed they had not handled the situation well, and she understood that patients are not interested in hearing about doctors' administrative foul-ups and frustrations. She also told me that my mammogram was basically fine, but they wanted me to come in for additional imaging of some calcifications. The head of the study had not been able to access my mammogram, but this physician could. I had my follow-up imaging that Wednesday and I was clear. The relief was incredible.

Questions remain, though. The MD running the study told me that the area of the cancer center where mammogram results were processed had closed unexpectedly, creating a four-day weekend. I was also told that the room containing the mammography results was locked and the doctor couldn't get it open. Surely staff, or someone, has master keys, though. If two radiologists were reading my mammogram in the morning, what happened between then and the remainder of the day that made the results of those readings unavailable? The doctor also said that getting my mammogram result required accessing a specific computer and she couldn't get that computer to give her my results. But health care systems have IT people working 24/7 to solve exactly this kind of problem. Finally, the physician told me that one of her two assistants had the day off. So many people were wanting a four-day weekend, I guess, but alas, my worry about cancer does not take a holiday.

Shane Sinclair et al. offer what they call "the first empirically based clinical model of compassion" in a 2016 article in the *Journal of Pain and Symptom Management*. Interestingly, they begin the article by quoting the American Medical Association's Code of Ethics, which affirms the importance of offering medical care with "compassion and respect for human dignity and rights." The problem, they state, is that although patients and clinicians know that compassionate care is needed, they are often unable to precisely define what it consists of. Patients in their study repeatedly defined compassionate care as clinicians evincing a "virtuous response to suffering," which included "knowing the person," making people the priority, and showing "beneficence." Most important of all, though, was what patients called "action," or manifesting compassion through behavior and activity. Action "was the quintessential feature of compassion." In particular, participants identified supererogatory acts, such as health care providers "going the extra mile" or when staff went "beyond the call of duty," as exemplars of compassionate action.

The failure of effective action by the staff involved in my mammogram result, and the excuses used to paper over that failure, hurt me. Problems that were either solvable or avoidable kept me from learning my mammography result in a timely way. The MD said she tried hard to get my results, but did she? I don't know. After I took to Twitter to complain, a different doctor read my scans, even though it was a weekend. That Saturday night, right after the head of radiology called me, Arthur and I met friends, a couple, for dinner. I described my mammography debacle and the positive end result, summarizing hopefully, "That's what happens when you go on Twitter." The husband replied, "No, Theresa. That's what happens when *you* go on Twitter."

It shouldn't be this way. Modern, technologically sophisticated health care does not have to be unfeeling, but it will be if the people using the technology do not prioritize feeling *for* patients. Cancer is scary, which makes mammography, or any kind of cancer screening, also scary. It was naïve of me to imagine that my needs would be elevated above the consternation of difficult computers, unexpectedly locked doors and staff on vacation, but I will not say it was wrong of me to want, even to expect, concern and thoughtfulness about my one-year mammogram.

If you're reading this and thinking that I ask for too much, that health care doesn't have time to consistently attend to patients' feelings, then consider this final piece of the story. While I was trying and failing to get mammography results from the doctor running the research study I participated in, my family practice physician, Dr. P, who told me I had breast cancer one day after my biopsies, was also trying to get my results, from Europe. Born overseas, he was visiting family, and took time out from that, disregarding the seven-hour time difference, to attempt to help.

His actions were supererogatory, and not a standard we could fairly hold all health care workers to, but in the moment, I felt his effort. He tried. He didn't succeed at getting the information I wanted, but he tried hard. He showed me that he cared.

THIRTY-SIX

Moving

WHEN WE MOVED to Pittsburgh in 2005, we sold our small house in Princeton, New Jersey, at the apex of the housing bubble. Homes in Pittsburgh were a lot cheaper than in Princeton, so we bought a three-story Victorian home on a tree-lined street. The third floor had three bedrooms and a bathroom for the kids. On the second floor we could now have a guest room and I would have a study to do my nursing school homework in. The front parlor was just the right size for the eight-foot-long grand piano that Arthur bought on eBay after inheriting some money from his grandmother. It was a lovely house, and yet I never fully felt at home there. It may have been more house than I wanted to take care of, though we have a lot of great memories from our time in it.

A year after my diagnosis, that third floor had been empty for an entire school year and the house really felt too big. Conrad would be moving to Michigan in the fall to get a PhD in economics and I knew that Miranda and Sophia would probably get their own apartment soon and would not return home for the summer. I actually dislike the relevant word here: downsize. It makes me think of people being turned into bugs. Downsizing also becomes complicated with an eight-foot grand piano. Let's just say that we wanted a smaller house with room for a pretty big piano.

We looked all over Pittsburgh, our indefatigably cheerful realtor insisting we view houses in a few of the city's neighborhoods. After several weeks, it all felt like too much. I was still chronically tired and maybe not quite ready to leave the home where we had mostly raised our kids. Then I got an automatic mailing from our realtor that included a few new houses. Clicking through them, I saw the house I wanted. Our realtor, JoAnne, had said we would know right away when we found the right place. She was right and we bought that house.

The new house was in a new neighborhood, so we picked up from our community of stately homes and near-perfect lawns in the East End of Pittsburgh and moved to Manchester, an integrated, more urban-feeling community on Pittsburgh's North Side. I love it here. People are friendly in a way I associate with growing up in Missouri, and downtown Pittsburgh is now close enough that it feels like we are really part of the city.

The neighborhood is wonderful, but the house was truly the draw. It is one side of a duplex, three stories tall, and was built of solid stone and red brick in 1892. The roof of the house had been literally falling in, and someone, we don't know who, transformed the rotting interior into a contemporary wonder. The first-floor staircase floats upwards, creating streaks of light between the slats of the stairs. An opening above the kitchen—technically an oculus—sends light from two second-story windows down into the kitchen workspace, and Arthur's and my bedroom has a huge window that lets in light all day due to its southern exposure. The circular staircase that ascends to the third floor makes a slatted pattern of light rectangles at night as it climbs upwards, giving the vibe of a film noir, without the gangsters, guns, and femme fatales. The bathroom doors are made of frosted glass to let in as much light as possible. JoAnne observed, "You like light," when we started looking at houses. She put into words what I'm not sure I could have, but I do like light. As a bonus, the house's open floor plan meant a grand piano would fit. In fact, there was already a piano in the house, albeit smaller than Arthur's.

We moved in right before Christmas of 2018. I bought a two-foot-high artificial tree and set it up on the hearth with a few ornaments. I don't remember much of that Christmas either, same as the year before, but it's a happy blur of unpacking and finding our rhythms in the new house, including where the light switches were. When people ask why we moved, I usually say it was time for a change, but I'm not sure I would have been galvanized to make this switch if I hadn't had cancer. Afterwards, I wanted to live in a whimsical house filled with light, and now I do.

THIRTY-SEVEN

Sue Larson

WHEN I FIRST heard Sue Larson's story, I didn't believe it. I was spending two weeks in Newnan, Georgia, in spring of 2019 as part of a writer's residency. I stayed in a small house that was included with the writing fellowship and worked on, well, this book. I also gave public talks and one of them was for a program in Newnan called "The Other Night School." The talks were collaboratively organized with the University of West Georgia's (UWG) English Department and Sue Larson was a regular attendee.

Before I arrived in Newnan, Sue told the UWG professor who organized "The Other Night School" a remarkable story that, as I said, I had a hard time believing. Upon learning that I was coming to Newnan, Sue read my book *The Shift: One Nurse, Twelve Hours, Four Patients' Lives* a month or so before my arrival. One of the four patients in the book—if you haven't read it, spoiler alert—has a perforated intestine, and it took longer than it should have for us, her medical team, to figure that out.

This is the story the professor told me. Soon after reading *The Shift*, Sue developed intense pain in her abdomen. She went to the hospital and the physicians and nurses there couldn't figure out what was wrong with her. Sue, who lives in Douglasville, Georgia (about twenty miles west of Atlanta) remembered the story of my patient in *The Shift* and told her doctor she had read "this book" that was relevant. A CT scan of her abdomen had been interpreted as normal, and Sue asked them to please recheck the scan. She said that at first they didn't take seriously her comment about a book she'd read that might help deduce the cause of her abdominal pain, but when she explained about the patient with the perforated intestine and a delayed diagnosis, they listened. The doctor rechecked Sue's CT scan, and—you know what's coming, right?—she had a perforated intestine.

The longer a perforation remains undetected and therefore untreated, the more time intestinal bacteria are inside the usually sterile space of the gut. A serious infection called peritonitis can develop. Patients can become septic, go into shock, and in the worst case die, but that happens over hours or days, not minutes. A perforation is a slow-motion medical emergency. Treatment has two parts: abdominal surgery to repair or remove the part of the colon that tore and may have died due to lack of good blood flow, and restoration or re-creation of a functioning gastrointestinal tract. For Sue, this meant connecting the healthy, nontorn part of her intestine to her abdomen and creating an opening for waste at the spot in her belly where the intestine joined up from inside.

In other words, Sue would now poop into a bag attached to the hole in her abdomen, called a stoma, from the word *stomach*. The new surgically created conduit for waste removal is called a colostomy and, in general, patients find colostomies difficult, but such details were far from my mind when I heard Sue's story. I could not believe my book helped save someone's life. *Really?* I asked. Then, close to the end of my visit, I met Sue Larson, the real still-alive Sue Larson. It was just before I spoke at "The Other Night School." We hugged, of course, and Sue, who is middle-aged with a friendly smile and shoulder-length blonde hair, gave me a card. Her husband showed me the passage from *The Shift* that got Sue correctly diagnosed and they asked me to sign her copy of my book and initial the passages. At that moment in *The Shift*, I'm doing a routine morning assessment of the patient with the pseudonym Sheila Fields. I listen to her belly with my stethoscope and wait to hear normal gurgling, except that I don't hear gurgling—I hear nothing. That's it. Human bellies are naturally loud when listened to with a stethoscope. A lack of intestinal bubbling may not indicate a serious problem, but it can.

Later that night, after my talk, when I had returned to the little house, I opened the card Sue gave me. Here is what she wrote:

Hi Theresa,

    There isn't enough room on here to tell you how grateful I am that you wrote this book. It's amazing how it all played out and I know God had a lot to do with it.

Chad told us about the book one night at class. That same night I went online and bought it. I read it and gave it to my husband to read. A week after he finished it, I end up in the hospital living it. Simply amazing!

. . . I truly think of you as an angel helping me through this.

The card Sue gave me has a drawing made with a few simple lines, of a young woman on a beach. Her face is barely in profile and she wears a loose white shift that makes her look sort of like an angel. In the sand she has written THANK YOU, followed by a heart symbol. The card itself is tactile, with patches of glitter giving the feel of sand, waves, and the shoreline in between.

My feelings about Sue and her experience are a jumble. Part of me feels I do not deserve her thanks, part of me thinks I do. "Sheila Fields's" story in *The Shift* is the story of a mistake. I wrote about my mistake—not pausing to think over what I did not hear in her belly—but there were errors of assessment up and down the line. Whoever evaluated her in the emergency department got caught up in her congenital blood disorder, which was ostensibly why she came to the hospital via ambulance, and ignored her abdomen. The intern and nurse on night shift failed to remark the quiet in her belly. It was the oncologist who ordered a CT scan around ten in the morning, "Just in case." Maybe he deserves the thanks. But then again, he didn't write my book—I did.

In my first draft of *The Shift*, I tried not to show my bungle with Sheila, my failure. I tried to write around it. It almost felt like I would die if I had to put what actually happened into words that *someone else*, maybe a lot of someone elses, would read. I really thought the shame would consume me, like a fire, like an unbearable pain. My editor—who's also the editor of this book—said about my attempt to hide what happened with Sheila, *This doesn't work*. She called out my feint, my sleight of hand. And I crept through that shame and pain to put the words down on paper, to write the passage that saved Sue's life, but also said to readers, *This is when I failed my patient. Right here. Read it here. Read about my failure here.*

Another time, another mistake, a much smaller one. I was working outpatient oncology at a different hospital than before. Sometimes we worked off orders that had been faxed in and were as a result hard to read. A patient was ordered a dose of an injectable steroid that was two or three times normal. At smaller doses we give the drug intravenously as a single injection. I wasn't sure about giving the larger dose the same way, but I didn't see anything in the order that indicated otherwise, so I drew up the injection and gave it to the patient. And then someone, I can't remember if it was me, saw a note on the side of the order that read, in small, uncertain handwriting that was very faint, "IV," and gave a time, fifteen minutes, I think.

I wanted the earth to open up and swallow me. I had given a drug IV push, in one single-shot dose, that was supposed to drip in. It felt like the worst thing I had ever done. To notify the physician who had ordered the drug, I found a phone tucked away in a recess on the floor, distant from the other nurses, and called. The doctor was calm and reassuring. I should watch for a possible drop in blood pressure, but probably my mix-up would make no difference at all. Huh. I thought the earth should crack apart and envelop me for that? I couldn't square my feelings and his reaction. I made a mistake, yes, but it made no difference.

Unfortunately, not all errors are so inconsequential, and making an error provokes intense anxiety because many of them are fatal. The number of deaths from medical errors in the U.S. is estimated to be 250,000 patients every year. *Every year.* And no one is doing much to change that, even when something as simple as a standardized medication order form would have meant I gave the ordered dose of steroid the right way. Caring for patients is a sacred duty; they trust us with their health and literally their lives. The patient should be every nurse's and doctor's North Star, but if our hospitals take errors, including deadly mistakes, for granted, the light from that star gets harder and harder to see. A dose of steroid given the wrong way is not too terrible. If a gaggle of clinicians miss the signs of a bowel perforation, which admittedly are not always easy to discern, the consequences are potentially severe. My patient Sheila Fields had some rough times in intensive care following her surgery, though she did go home in the end.

Sue, though, Sue did great. Ileostomies and colostomies can be reversed and Sue, it turns out, was a good candidate for a reversal. Her G.I. tract has been restored and she is doing well in Douglasville, GA, working, and gardening and playing tennis again. Sue felt cared for, was cared for, because her doctor listened to her. That listening, done well, made all the difference in Sue's care and probably saved her life.

THIRTY-EIGHT

Two Afternoons in Hospice

THERE WERE GOOD moments in the hospice job that I returned to after cancer. One family, Orthodox Jews, lived in Pittsburgh's Squirrel Hill neighborhood and I'd been their nurse once a few months before. The patient was an older man living in his daughter's house. For that visit, he didn't comprehend much of what I said, and I remember getting cues from the daughter not to ask about certain things. One of them was pain, because he would say that his entire body hurt, but never complained if he wasn't asked.

The patient's daughter told me his back did hurt from an old injury that had nothing to do with his hospice diagnosis. He sat watching television, scrunched down into a thick-cushioned couch that seemed to swallow him. My back would hurt if I sat like that all day, I thought, probably irrelevantly, but that was where he always sat when the family watched television, and they were watching congressional hearings on C-SPAN during my visit. I didn't feel too helpful since every question I asked got swatted away by the daughter. I felt like they didn't really want me there, and truth be told, the patient seemed fine, all things considered. He was breathing and sleeping with no problems. His appetite was OK. The daughter clarified that his back only hurt when he stood up and sat down, making it hard to treat since it was intermittent. Also, his knees bothered him a little bit, his daughter explained, but not so much that they interfered with his living his fairly constrained life.

Fast forward several months, and the patient was close to death. I got to the house, one of those great old Pittsburgh houses with an impressive front door, and the daughter let me in. The front entry hall had beautiful wood paneling and a large staircase with a landing in the middle, most of its width taken up with a lift chair. The daughter directed me upstairs and I followed after. Her father was in the first bedroom on the right, just at the top of the stairs. The room where I'd seen him before, where the TV had been, was next door and much larger. This room was smaller, more intimate. The patient lay in a hospital bed that hospice had supplied. He looked comfortable and didn't respond to me or anyone else who came into the room.

Three granddaughters came in soon after I arrived, one very upset, one calm, the other analytical. They had many questions and I talked with them about how to best care for someone at the end of his life. I said to give morphine if the patient needed it, but if he looked comfortable, they could leave him be. I told them to observe his face closely to make sure he had no pain. As people die, their facial expressions tend to become more fixed, and I encouraged the granddaughters to check for squinching up of the eyes or tightening around the patient's mouth—those might be signs of increasing pain. Then I talked about how people die, stressing that one system after another will fail, but predicting the order is difficult. One patient will stop producing urine, indicating kidney failure, while another will display deep blue mottling of the legs, suggesting the heart is not pumping oxygenated blood as well as it needs to. I explained that when many people get close to death they develop apneic breathing: they stop breathing for several seconds, then start up again. If the apneic period lasts long enough, the people in the room think the patient has died, only to have the patient start breathing again with a snort, a suck, sometimes a gasp. It can be very hard to be in a room with someone having apneic breathing and I told them that it was important to take breaks.

I don't know how much of it sunk in. I'm not sure how much of all that I would have understood in my teens and early twenties. Death, like aging, can feel so far away to the young. The granddaughters were satisfied enough with my answers that they left the room, leaving the daughter and me alone. Two simple desk chairs were set up next to each other in front of the bedroom window, facing the bed. The daughter was already sitting in one of them and I sat down in the other to talk. We talked about her husband's work schedule and her son's driving lessons. She asked me about my kids and I described the twins and Conrad, off in Ann Arbor, Michigan, for graduate school.

It was a pleasant spring afternoon outside and I remember a breeze coming in through the window. We chatted for a while, with no change in the patient's condition, and then I said I should go. It was my last visit of the day and the patient needed a refill on his pain medication so I would take care of that. I also had follow-up phone calls to make, notes to send to the regular nurses of the patients I saw that day (remember, I was "casual"), and a special note about this patient, since he was in the middle of what we called "actively dying."

Ordering a refill of narcotic pain medication for a patient on home hospice is always a multistep process. This patient was on a fentanyl patch. It released medication slowly through his skin and the hospice had set up administrative barriers to easy refills on fentanyl patches because fentanyl was, in their view, expensive. The refill process began with my calling the MD to get an order. Opioid prescriptions, unlike those for other drugs, cannot simply be renewed—a brand new order is necessary. Next, I called our pharmacy benefits manager (PBM), which meant I left a voicemail message and waited for someone to call me back. PBMs are third-party companies that "administer" prescriptions for health care companies, and they have incredible power to influence, and sometimes dictate, prescribing practices. The PBM authorized most medications without any extra steps, but fentanyl patches needed a manager's approval before the PBM would release the fentanyl order to our hospice pharmacy. I called the pharmacy and told them the drug needed to be delivered to the patient's home that night. Patches last for seventy-two hours and his was going to run out that evening. If the medication wasn't a rush order, I could have had the PBM mail the medication to the patient's home, since mailing is cheaper than home delivery, and evening or after-hours delivery of a drug, which this patient would need, was frowned upon due to the expense. The rules sound commonsensical, but needs in health care sometimes subvert common sense.

I told the PBM that the patient had no more fentanyl patches and without them would be in extreme pain from end-stage cancer. I couldn't get my manager on the phone, so I left a voicemail and also sent an email. The hospice administrator had quickly faxed the physician order for fentanyl to the pharmacy, but the pharmacy would not move on it because my manager had not called the PBM so the PBM could not verify the order with the pharmacy. PBMs, by the way, supposedly exist to save money, and since I wasn't being paid fairly for my time, they might have in this case, but imagine if my time had been appropriately valued. Back at home, finishing up my work for the day, I made a phone call for a different patient, sent another email, and then called back the PBM, who called me back and told me that my manager still hadn't approved the fentanyl order. I called the pharmacy, where I also had to leave a message, telling them that the medication absolutely had to go out tonight. When they called back, they hemmed and hawed a bit. They would do their best, but couldn't guarantee an evening delivery since they were still waiting for the PBM's approval and they would mostly close up shop, except for deliveries, in an hour or so.

I decided to stop calling the PBM and the pharmacy, implicitly demanding that they do something they were not allowed to do. I had finished up my other paperwork, so I left another voicemail for my manager and sent her another email, and then quit. That night I lay awake in bed with a sick feeling in my stomach, worrying that the poor patient was suffering through the night because, in the moment, controlling costs mattered more than controlling a dying patient's pain.

The next afternoon I saw the Squirrel Hill patient again. He had received the fentanyl patch refill the night before. *Unbelievable*, I thought. Spending two hours alternately bullying and begging people over the phone can produce results. I had gone back to the patient's house because he was actively dying. That meant he would receive one visit every day, and more if needed. He appeared very much the way he had the day before, maybe a little more drawn into himself and breathing a little more slowly. The daughter and I again sat down in the chairs facing the bed and she said they removed the chair lift yesterday after I left because they knew he wouldn't use it again. "Oh," I said, explaining that the staircase had seemed wider to me, but I couldn't put my finger on why.

Somehow talk turned to the shooting the October before at the nearby Tree of Life synagogue. The shooting made the national news and brought then-President Trump to Pittsburgh. People led vigils outside for weeks afterwards. I know because we lived only three blocks away and sometimes when I walked our dog at night I would stop by. The patient's daughter told me details I hadn't known: that Orthodox Jews don't take personal identification into synagogue and the bodies were so mangled that the victims were difficult to identify. Also, Jewish law stipulates that all parts of a body must be buried, requiring careful collection by trained volunteers of the victims' blood from the synagogue floor. The one victim I knew, just a little, had previously prepared bodies with the same volunteers who were now gathering his blood. He was a decent man and a very compassionate doctor. I couldn't reconcile what I knew of him with how his life had ended.

The daughter and I talked then, as we had the day before, about the funeral rites she wanted observed for her father. Hospice nurses often wash a patient's body after death, but in the Orthodox Jewish tradition, a ritual washing of the dead is done by trained members of the community, similar to those who cleaned up the victims' blood at Tree of Life. It is difficult to know which hospice nurse will come to a patient's pronouncement because when the patient will die is uncertain. That evening I put a note in several places in the chart, all in caps, specifying that no one from hospice should wash the body. When the patient died a few days later, his regular nurse emailed me specially to say that the Orthodox practices had been observed. It felt like I had done a *mitzvah*, a good deed.

That second afternoon I also sat with the daughter in front of the bedroom window and felt the same warm spring breeze come in. The patient was leaving the world so peacefully; there was little for me to do clinically. The daughter was not distraught. She did not need my emotional support. But still I sat, and we talked of this and that, until a fair amount of time had passed and I felt the pull of those notes I still needed to write, those phone calls I had to make.

Both days I left feeling satisfied about a job well done, and I know I would never have felt that way before my diagnosis and treatment, back when I delivered care according to a more or less Maslovian hierarchy of needs. Pain would always get my attention, and shortness of breath was very important, too. That would be followed, in order, by vomiting or other GI distress, wounds and skin breakdown, eating and sleeping, and anything else physically wrong. Emotional pain—of the patient or members of the family—traveled on its own separate, but important, track.

But sitting and talking? About kids, or why the daughter bought the house she did (it was a good story), or what her own daughters were up to? No one ever told me how much that could matter. How much someone in a difficult place might want not support, but companionship, a moment to feel ordinary, to be ordinary, a moment to remember that one's whole life was not the totality of a father dying, or being a woman with breast cancer.

THIRTY-NINE

The New Road

I DIDN'T WORK many night shifts on home hospice, but sometimes I volunteered when needed. The shifts were unpredictable. One night I wasn't called out at all and I woke up at seven the next morning reaching for my work phone in a panic, sure I had slept through something important. But I hadn't—there were no nighttime emergencies.

Another night I was out for literally the entire night. My evening started with a pronouncement and I had to find a house up a twisty suburban road in the dark in pouring rain. I got two new calls while I was still busy at that house. There was another pronouncement, this time at a nursing home. Then I went off on a wild goose chase at a different nursing home. They called in saying they had an emergency, but when I arrived, all the doors were locked, no one answered the phone, and no people could be seen through the glass doors in front of the brightly lit, unstaffed front desk. I thought briefly about walking around the building and knocking on any lit windows I found, but decided that would not end well.

Another night, I had only one call. It came around two in the morning. I had no trouble waking up to answer the phone, put on my uniform, brush my teeth, and make sure my hair wasn't a mess. I grabbed my bag next to the front door and went. I had a name, an address, and a problem to fix: the patient's intravenous pain pump had run out of medication and the family couldn't figure out how to replace the empty cartridge with a new one. The patient had cancer and was likely in agony. A patient's pump should never run out. Never. Values-based care is a new idea in health care, intended to determine "value" by comparing the economic costs of treatment with what we euphemistically call "good outcomes." How, though, does one assess the value of relieving a patient's pain versus the cost of not doing that? We need a metric for "lack of compassion."

There's very little traffic at two a.m., which makes driving easy, and I felt thankful for that. When I got off the highway, taking the exit for the patient's suburb, I saw that the road ahead was brightly lit and workers in hardhats were milling around it next to big machines. Cones were set up on the left side of the road, and the right side was outlined by a string of flagged posts connected by thick rope. The crew was repaving the road and had just finished the lane I would drive on. As I edged onto the fresh asphalt, I could feel its smoothness under my tires. I thought, *I am the first person to drive on this new pavement.* I would never have had that experience if I had not been called out that night, to that place, at that time. The road continued, feeling frictionless, until I got to the turnoff and left it behind. After a few more turns, I arrived at the patient's two-story colonial, its wood shutters just distinguishable against the house's lighter walls. The entire street was dark.

A middle-aged man met me at the door and led me into a first-floor room. When I saw the patient, I understood the situation. A young woman, emaciated, with large, wounded eyes, stared at me out of a mound of pillows and blankets that surrounded her on a bed. A middle-aged woman sat on the edge of the bed, making noises like the soft coos of a dove. The patient was this couple's daughter. I was not making a nighttime visit to an elderly dying aunt, mother, grandmother. That would be sad, of course, but this—this was tragic, awful. Their faces were lined with worry and she looked at me with unexpressed yearning. I hadn't looked up the patient on my computer before I left because I wanted to get to the house as quickly as possible. I knew what I had to do during the visit, but I was unprepared for the anguish of the situation.

The father gave me a new cartridge for his daughter's pain pump. Every patient on a pump always has at least one spare cartridge in the house. As the father handed over the cartridge, I realized he was saying something to me. He was apologizing for pulling me out of my bed, or wherever he thought I had been, and into their house in the middle of the night. He was apologizing for not being able to replace the cassette filled with pain medication himself.

"This is my work," I said. I tried to sound neutral but affirming. His apology struck me as obscene. I wanted to apologize to him, to show regret that his daughter, who looked roughly the age of my daughters, was dying of cancer and we had let her pain pump run dry. I could not imagine the horror of having to sit, helpless, while my dying child experienced the pain of terminal cancer, waiting for a nurse from far away to arrive. I wished I could heal her with my hands, or at least snap my fingers and make their memories of this terrible night go away. But I couldn't do either.

Instead, I did my job. The pumps made for home use are small, a little thicker and more oblong than a standard paperback book. Every pump has a small screen and I checked it to make sure the pump was working and to verify that the narcotic cartridge was empty. Replacing the cartridge requires a special key that every hospice nurse carries, but this family had a key, too, and the father gave me theirs before I asked for it. The key allows the old cartridge to release and I took it off, connected the tubing on the new cartridge to the pump, and locked it back up, which takes some doing because the cartridge has to be held tightly in place for the key to work. The patient's father and mother watched me intently, standing at the side of their daughter's bed. I entered the new volume of medication into the pump's memory and rechecked the programmed dose with the ordered dose printed on the new cartridge. I would double-check the numbers against the patient's electronic chart, but before I did that, the most important part of the whole process needed to happen: "Give yourself a bolus," I told the patient.

She held up a small plastic tube with a red button on top. It connected to the pump via a thick wire and the pump connected to her body through thin intravenous tubing attached to the port in her chest. When she pressed the button, I saw the fluid in the tubing move up while the pump made a low mechanical sound. She closed her eyes and lay back on her pillows. Relief—for both of us, but much more for her. The pump gave her a steady dose of pain medication and she could give herself an additional dose—a bolus—when she needed it.

The mother left the room, but the father remained by the side of the bed, watching. I took off my latex gloves, squirted my hands with hand sanitizer and rubbed it in, then checked my laptop to verify that the dose settings on the patient's pump matched the physician's order in the computer. Normally I would chat a bit to see if the family needed anything else or if there were other issues to address, but the circumstances seemed beyond chat and it was three in the morning. Everyone in the house ought to sleep, if they could.

Before I left, I tried to make the patient's father understand that I was glad to be there and he needn't apologize for calling a nurse in at night. We stood in the foyer of the house, where the only light came through the door of his daughter's room. I do not know if he heard me. He seemed mentally far away, distracted by the coming devastation of his daughter's death.

Then I picked up my bag, walked to the car, and left. In Ernest Hemingway's *The Sun Also Rises*, the main character, Jake Barnes, says, "It is awfully easy to be hard-boiled about everything in the daytime, but at night it is another thing."

ANOTHER NEW ROAD: in June of 2021, as I was finishing this book, I stopped taking Tamoxifen. I didn't quit the drug impulsively because I was sick of the side effects—I switched from Tam to Arimidex, the other kind of medication for breast cancer prevention, called an aromatase inhibitor. In general, breast cancer patients who have not gone through menopause take Tamoxifen, and women who are postmenopausal take aromatase inhibitors (called AIs). A blood test showed low enough estrogen levels that we could assume I was done with menopause. My hope was that I would feel more like myself on Arimidex than I did on Tamoxifen, but I worried about making the switch before my full five years on Tam were up, wondering if a "the devil you know" approach was best.

My medical oncologist told me that it's impossible to predict how any one person will respond to AIs, but despite not knowing how Arimidex would affect *me*, I started it early. The side-effect profile of both drugs is very similar in terms of fatigue and brain fog. Aromatase inhibitors can also cause joint pain and lead to increased bone loss and osteoporosis, putting patients at risk of fractures. Two weeks after I started Arimidex, though, my tiredness, which had felt like a heavy oversized coat I wore everywhere I went, lessened significantly. It isn't gone, but it no longer rules my life. During that same time, my Tamoxifen-related brain fog evaporated. I have more hot flashes on Arimidex than I did on Tam, but getting my brain back is worth it. I may be sweaty, but I can think.

For the first time since my diagnosis, I stepped out from cancer's long shadow and felt able to envision a postcancer life. I will still have yearly mammograms, checkups, and a pill to take every day, as well as the occasional stabbing pain at the site of my lumpectomy scar. But fear of cancer, which is to say, the fear of dying, would become part of my past, not my present, and not an overwhelming worry for my future. I would stand in the sunshine, feel it warm my face, and understand that I was still fully alive.

I OFTEN THINK back to that nighttime visit to the young cancer patient whose father was so apologetic for calling a nurse out in the middle of the night. After I left the patient's house and turned onto the main road leading to the highway, I saw that the work crew I had seen on my way to the house was still paving, and their neon yellow vests shone in the bright lights that illuminated the road. It was summer and they all wore short sleeves, trying to stay cool as they worked in the still warm night air. I had the air-conditioning on in the car, maintaining a comfortable temperature despite the heat outside. For the rest of my solitary drive home, and even to this day, I kept those images—of hard work in the middle of the night, of an oasis of light and color amid the darkness, and of the smooth new road—fresh in the forefront of my mind.

Epilogue

BEING A CANCER patient exposed me to the cracks in U.S. health care in a new and painful way, and I could not figure out how best to adapt to that. As a nurse, I told myself that if the system failed patients, I could make up for it by working harder, better, longer. Sometimes that was true—as in the two hours spent trying to order a fentanyl patch—and sometimes it wasn't. As a patient I learned that too often the question is not *if* the system will fail us, but *when?*

I also have to admit that any one person giving 120 percent to the job cannot balance out work practices focused on profits and squeezing every last bit of effort from staff who only want to do good. How to fix that? We need some form of universal health care. Requiring that all health-care facilities be not-for-profit would make a big difference, too, as would eliminating the electronic paperwork demands that terribly burden clinical staff. The mandate of health care should be *caring*.

Almost exactly two years after my diagnosis of breast cancer, I quit home hospice and began teaching as a part-time faculty member at the University of Pittsburgh School of Nursing. Working with students felt right, but a master's degree in nursing is a requirement in Pennsylvania (and many other states) for teaching in a nursing school. I chose not to pursue that degree, which meant I had to resign. I had started a Clinical Nurse Leader program, but the degree felt more like a professional hoop than something I wanted to complete for its own sake. I also realized I didn't want to be in school, no matter the subject.

For the time being then, I'm a writer, and I'm still striving to understand everything I learned about health care as a patient. A sense of a more complete understanding came to me this past fall, when Arthur and I visited Chincoteague Island, Virginia. I first learned about Chincoteague as a kid from reading the book *Misty of Chincoteague*, which is about a pony, not a person. My mom took my brother and me there for summer vacation and I immediately loved the island. Arthur and I took our kids in turn when they were school-age, and we all still keep going even though the kids are grown up. Visiting Chincoteague usually means spending time on two islands: Chincoteague, of course, and Assateague, which is oceanside and separated by a bay from Chincoteague. Assateague traverses the Maryland–Virginia border and the Virginia portion of Assateague is a wildlife refuge, home to the famous (to some) wild ponies. (I do not know why the ponies on Assateague are called the Chincoteague ponies—perhaps because of the *Misty of Chincoteague* book.) The wonder of Assateague is that no development is allowed there, so the beaches are nothing but beach. No towering hotels or shop-lined boardwalks compromise the deep pleasure of sand, sky, and sea.

Why we visited a beach town in November is a long story, but we did, renting a small one-bedroom house located right on the bay that separates Chincoteague and Assateague. The house had a screened-in porch and on a few days it was warm enough to sit on the porch and read, drink my tea, and watch the occasional small boat go by. A couple times I spotted a hawk circling over the trees of Assateague. The island was so close to our house that the dark green of the trees stood out against the surrounding light blue sky and dark blue water.

On Chincoteague, Arthur and I had seen deer and we'd wondered where they came from—surely not the highway and bridge connecting the Virginia mainland to the island. One afternoon I was sitting on the porch and saw a deer standing on the shoal between our house and Assateague Island. This narrow strip of land in the bay was covered in marsh grass, but low tide revealed a sandbar that I could see from my chair. As I watched, the deer took a few steps out onto the sand, then kept walking into the water, lowering itself into the bay until it was completely submerged except for its head, which barely bobbed as it swam across the water towards me. Tall reeds prevented me from seeing it rise in the marsh just south of our house and climb out onto dry land, but I had learned that deer traveled between the islands by swimming. I didn't even know deer swam.

What is the lesson here? The deer is me, the patient, stuck out in the middle of the bay, diagnosed with breast cancer. I made it to dry ground by plunging in like the deer, and going through treatment. I climbed out on the other side, cancer-free as far as I know. Not whole, not yet a survivor, but recovered enough.

Not everyone will find this story inspiring. Some people even hate deer. But the thing about the deer is this: it didn't hesitate. It knew its way and it was elegant, graceful. It was one deer, but its singularity of purpose spoke to me in a metaphysical way, by which I mean with a power greater than the sum of the experience might suggest. That is healing. That is what compassion can accomplish. The deer stepped off the sandy shoal, put its hoof in the cold salt water, and never paused.

My treatment was not smooth like the deer's swim appeared to be. Making things easy for patients is not a goal of our health care system. Unlike the deer, my head jerked up and down as I struggled, as if I were treading water and getting nowhere, as if I had been thrown in and told to "sink or swim," as if I couldn't fully figure out how to get to the dry ground on the other side.

But it doesn't have to be that way. Treatment can be imbued with kindness and compassion so that caring for others feels like the act of grace that it is. We who do the caring can be as compassionate with each other as we are to patients. The system can guarantee everyone the care they need, no matter the color of their skin or the content of their bank account.

If we do these things, patients will not feel alone as they step into the water, take that life-saving plunge, swim, and in the end come out onto dry ground, if at all possible, healed.

ACKNOWLEDGMENTS

THANKS TO JILL Kneerim, my agent, friend, compass, and cheerleader. Surely Jill knows how fabulous she is, but I love that I get to put it in print in this book. A day of amazing good fortune first brought me together with Amy Gash, my editor at Algonquin Books, and now I have the pleasure of working with Amy on a second book; despite my cancer diagnosis, that makes me feel lucky. Amy gave me the idea of writing the book as a series of short chapters—"gemlike" in my aspirational description, and the key to making it work. Thanks also to Michael McKenzie and his publicity team at Algonquin. Michael somehow manages to make book promotion fun, which is not easy.

Many people helped me during my treatment. Thanks especially to Jill for the cupcakes, Nancy for the pizza and pedicure, Lisa for Thai food, Shannon for the card that made me feel brave, and Fred S. for the card that made me feel loved. Thanks to Julia for the frequent phone calls, Beth for common sense and laughter, and Josh for being an awesome physician and friend. If I haven't named you, it's only because the list would get too long. Any gesture, no matter how small, was appreciated. I tend to go to ground when the world seems dark, but so many of you found me there and offered cheering words, helpful conversation, hugs. There was even a beautiful orchid, sent to the house by someone I barely know.

A shoutout to Billie Holiday's "Don't Explain." The song is about infidelity, which isn't relevant to this book or my life, but I focused on that phrase "don't explain" to guide me as I wrote. Another shoutout to my daughter, Miranda Kosowsky, who, finding herself at loose ends during the summer of COVID-19, did some research for the book. And a special thanks to friends Julia Judish (who called regularly) and Mari Schindele, who read the book in draft and made it better than it would have been otherwise. Elliott Mower has been my social media and IT guru through two books now, and I honestly couldn't do that part of authorship without him. Finally, I made a solid start on the book during a two-week artist-in-residence stint in Newnan, Georgia, in the spring of 2019. Thanks to the Fred R. and Nell W. Blackwell Testamentary Trust, the Newnan Artist-in-Residence Program, and the School of the Arts at the University of West Georgia for making that two-week stay possible.

The tragedy of cancer, for me, would have been leaving my kids without a mother. I am so glad it has not come to that. Nor will I leave my husband without a wife. Thank you all for being the wonderful people you are and enriching my life in ways that heretofore seemed unimaginable. I hope to be around for a long time.

REFERENCES

Chapter 3 "Bob & Wendy"

Mark Kurlansky, *Cod: A Biography of the Fish That Changed the World* (New York: Penguin Books, 1997).

Chapter 5 "Storytelling"

Leslie Marmon Silko, "Tony's Story," *Storyteller* (New York: Seaver Books, 1981), 123–9.

Chapter 6 "An Ideal Patient"

Beth Lown, Julie Rosen, and John Martilla, "An Agenda for Improving Compassionate Care: A Survey Shows About Half of Patients Say Such Care Is Missing," *Health Affairs*, September 2011, 1772.

Hannah B. Wild, "There's No Algorithm for Empathy," *Health Affairs*, February 2020, available online at https://doi.org/10.1377/hlthaff.2019.00571.

Chapter 7 "What We Talk About When We Talk About Amputation"

Ziad Obermeyer et al., "Dissecting Racial Bias in an Algorithm Used to Manage the Health of Populations, *Science*, October 25, 2019, 4.

Chapter 12 "Balance"

"Crime in the City of Pittsburgh Categorized for Uniform Crime Reporting (UCR), 2010 through April 2021." Last updated 4/30/2021, available online at https://tableau .alleghenycounty.us/t/PublicSite/views/CJ_UCR_PGH _8-22-17_v3/Home_1?iframeSizedToWindow=true&%3 Aembed=y&%3AshowAppBanner=false&%3Adisplay _count=no&%3AshowVizHome=no&%3Aorigin=viz _share_link.

American Cancer Society, "Cancer Disparities in the Black Community," available online at https://www.cancer.org /about-us/what-we-do/health-equity/cancer-disparities-in -the-black-community.html.

Chapter 14 "Not on the List"

Stephen Trzeciak and Anthony Mazzarelli, *Compassionomics: The Revolutionary Scientific Evidence That Caring Makes a Difference* (Pensacola, FL: Studer Group, 2019), 63.

Chapter 15 "Theresa in Cancerland"

Leslie Jamison, "I Used to Insist I Didn't Get Angry. Not Anymore. On Female Rage," *New York Times Magazine*, January 17, 2018, available online at https://www.nytimes .com/2018/01/17/magazine/i-used-to-insist-i-didnt-get -angry-not-anymore.html.

Chapter 17 "Nature/Nurture"

Audre Lorde, "Today Is Not the Day," *The Marvelous Arithmetics of Distance: Poems 1987–1992* (New York: W.W. Norton & Company, 1993), 57.

Chapter 18 "Chemo: Yes or No"

Michel Foucault, *The Birth of the Clinic: An Archaeology of Medical Perception*, trans. A. M. Sheridan Smith (New York: Random House, 1994), 8 and 83.

Chapter 24 "Tam"

Hongchao Pan et al., "20-Year Risks of Breast-Cancer Recurrence after Stopping Endocrine Therapy at 5 Years," *New England Journal of Medicine*, November 2017, 1843.

Chapter 25 "Tam, Continued"

Audre Lorde, *The Cancer Journals* (San Francisco: Aunt Lute Books, 1980), 9.

Chapter 27 "On the Side"

National Comprehensive Cancer Network, "NCCN Guidelines Version 2.2018 Cancer Related Fatigue," available online at https://blog.summit-education.com/wp-content/uploads/NCCN-Profesional-Guidelines-CRF.pdf.

Julienne E. Bower et al., "Cytokine Genetic Variations and Fatigue among Patients with Breast Cancer," *Journal of Clinical Oncology*, May 1, 2013, 1656–61.

César Fernández-de-las-Peñas et al., "Catechol-O-methyltransferase Genotype (Val158met) Modulates Cancer-Related Fatigue and Pain Sensitivity in Breast Cancer Survivors," *Breast Cancer Research Treatment*, 2012, 405–12.

Chapter 28 "Figures of Speech"

Susan Sontag, *Illness as Metaphor* and *AIDS and Its Metaphors* (New York: Picador, 1990), 182–3.

Barbara Ehrenreich, *Bright-Sided: How Positive Thinking Is Undermining America* (New York: Henry Holt & Company, 2009), 33.

Samantha Artiga, Kendal Orgera, and Olivia Pham, "Disparities in Health and Health Care: Five Key Questions and Answers," Kaiser Family Foundation Issue Brief, March 4, 2020, available online at https://www.kff.org /racial-equity-and-health-policy/issue-brief/disparities-in -health-and-health-care-five-key-questions-and-answers/.

American Cancer Society, "Impact of Attitudes and Feelings on Cancer," December 4, 2020, available online at https://www.cancer.org/treatment/survivorship-during-and -after-treatment/coping/attitudes-and-feelings-about -cancer.html.

Stephen Trzeciak and Anthony Mazzarelli, *Compassionomics: The Revolutionary Scientific Evidence That Caring Makes a Difference* (Pensacola, FL: Studer Group, 2019), xv.

Kevin R. Binning et al., "Changing Social Contexts to Foster Equity in College Science Courses: An Ecological-Belonging Intervention," *Psychological Science, 2020*, 1059.

Chapter 35 "One-Year Mammogram"

Shane Sinclair et al., "Compassion in Health Care: An Empirical Model," *The Journal of Pain and Symptom Management*, 2016, 193–203.

ADDITIONAL READING

I FOUND SUSAN Love, MD's book on breast cancer, aptly entitled *Dr. Susan Love's Breast Book*, helpful as a comprehensive resource for breast cancer patients, though I dipped into it sparingly, as I did with all writing about breast cancer. Multiple editions are available.

If interested, the books listed below are the best I've read on the profiteering and illogic of American health care. Each provides excellent analysis and in different ways shows that the biggest problem of the U.S. health care system may be that it isn't a system at all.

Stephen Brill, *America's Bitter Pill: Money, Politics, Backroom Deals, and the Fight to Fix Our Broken Healthcare System* (New York: Random House, 2015).

Mike Magee, *Code Blue: Inside America's Medical Industrial Complex* (New York: Atlantic Monthly Press, 2019).

T. R. Reid, *The Healing of America: A Global Quest for Better, Cheaper, and Fairer Health Care* (New York: Penguin Books, 2009).

Elisabeth Rosenthal, *An American Sickness: How Healthcare Became Big Business and How You Can Take It Back* (New York: Penguin Books, 2017).